STRESS AND THE HEART

Mechanisms, Measurements, and Management

by

Robert S. Eliot, M.D., F.A.C.C.

Director, The Cardiovascular Institute
Swedish Medical Center
Denver, Colorado

With contributions by

Daniel Baker, Ph.D.
Jeffrey L. Boone, M.D.
W. Thomas Boyce, M.D.
James C. Buell, M.D.
C. Wayne Callaway, M.D.

Anne M. Garland, R.N.
Gregory A. Harshfield, P.D.
David R. Long, M.D.
Hugo Morales-Ballejo, M.D.
Thomas Sawyer, Ph.D.

Elizabeth Yaeger, M.D.

Futura Publishing Co., Inc.
Mount Kisco, New York
1988

Library of Congress Cataloging-in-Publication Data

Eliot, Robert S.
Stress and the heart.

Includes bibliographies and index.
1. Heart—Diseases. 2. Stress (Psychology)
I. Title. [DNLM: 1. Cardiovascular Diseases.
2. Stress, Psychological. WG 100 E42s]
RC682.9.E45   1988   616.1'2   87-30307
ISBN 0-87993-317-8

Copyright © 1988
Futura Publishing Company, Inc.

Published by:
Futura Publishing Company, Inc.
295 Main Street
Mount Kisco, New York 10549

LC#: 87-30307
ISBN#: 0-87993-317-8

Contributors

Daniel Baker, Ph.D.
Executive Director for Health
  Services
Canyon Ranch Resort
Tucson, Arizona

Jeffrey L. Boone, M.D.
Clinic Director
Cardiovascular Institute
Swedish Medical Center
Denver, Colorado

W. Thomas Boyce, M.D.
Associate Professor, Pediatrics
University of California
San Francisco, California

James C. Buell, M.D.
Associate Professor of Cardiology
  and Chief of Cardiology
Health Sciences Center, School of
  ˊMedicine
Texas Tech University
Lubbock, Texas

C. Wayne Callaway, M.D.
Director, Center for Clinical
  Nutrition
George Washington University
  Medical Center
Washington, D.C.

**Anne M. Garland, R.N., B.S.N.,
  C.S.E.**
Educator and Consultant
Cardio Concepts, Inc.
Litchfield Park, Arizona

Gregory A. Harshfield, Ph.D.
Associate Professor of Internal
  Medicine
Charles R. Drew Postgraduate
  Medical School
King/Drew Medical Center
Los Angeles, California

David R. Long, M.D., F.A.C.C.
Director of Medical Services
Occupational Health Network
Phoenix, Arizona

**Hugo Morales-Ballejo, M.D.,
  F.A.C.C.**
Director of Clinical Research
Cardiovascular Institute
Swedish Medical Center
Denver, Colorado

Thomas Sawyer, Ph.D.
Director of Behavioral Medicine
National Center of Preventive
  and Stress Medicine
St. Luke's Heart Lung Center
Phoenix, Arizona

Elizabeth Yaeger, M.D.
Chief of Affective Disorder Clinic
Mental Health Annex, Maricopa
  County Medical Center
Phoenix, Arizona

Acknowledgments

Many friends and colleagues have provided support and inspiration for this text. I would particularly like to thank the Monsour Medical Foundation and The International Stress Foundation without whose support this book would not have been possible.

Important input was provided by my collaborators and colleagues: Doctors Dan Baker, Jeffrey Boone, Tom Boyce, James C. Buell, C. Wayne Callaway, Gregory A. Harshfield, David Long, Hugo Morales-Ballejo, Thomas Sawyer, and Elizabeth Yaeger; also Anne Garland, Jeff Smolin, and Karen Woodhouse.

The review of an early version of the book by Dr. Benjamin M. Kaplan helped greatly in determining the tone and focus of the text.

Reprints and personal communications supplied valuable material incorporated into the text. In this regard I wish to thank Doctors Theodore M. Dembroski, Warren Grundfest, William Kannel, Mark McKinney, Dean Ornish, S. Leonard Syme, and Stephen M. Weiss.

Much of chapter 8 ("Use of Impedance for Hypertension") appeared earlier in *Illustrated Medicine*. We thank the publisher, Wynwood Publishing, Inc. for allowing us to reprint this material.

The interpretations, coordination, and verification of the information supplied by me and others was the task of my medical editor, Esther Adler. I am grateful for her skilled and dedicated work.

Helping me to find the time to make this book possible were my able assistants, Joann Hall, Marilyn Miller, and Carmen Smith. Last but not least, my dear wife, Phyllis, who for more than three decades, always provided the love, understanding, and moral support that keeps my stress manageable.

Table of Contents

SECTION I
Mechanisms Linking Stress to Cardiovascular Damage

SECTION II
Diagnosis and Evaluation

SECTION III
Management

SECTION IV
Special Problems

OVERVIEW

The world's literature concerning the role of lifestyle, behavior, and stress in heart disease has burgeoned in the last five years. According to Dr. Stephen Weiss, director of the Behavioral Medicine Branch of the National Heart, Lung, and Blood Institute, between fifty and seventy-five billion dollars of the nation's four-hundred billion dollar health bill are spent for stress-linked illnesses. Indeed two-thirds of all visits to family physicians are related to stress-linked illnesses, and with regard to new coronary events, the standard risk factors account only for somewhat less than 50%.

For a long time, theory and practice went far beyond knowledge and technology. However, advances in pathophysiology have provided new insights, and modern biotechnology now permits a more comprehensive evaluation of the metabolic, endocrine, and immunologic impact of stress. Computerized data processing has greatly enhanced this development through the ease of tabulating relationships and bodily effects.

We now know the consequences of "stress" more precisely than we know the definition of it. Stress may be viewed as the body's response to any real or imagined events perceived as requiring some adaptive response and/or producing strain. This allows us then to differentiate between stress (the internally mediated adaptive response) and stressors (the stimuli). While stressors can be physical or mental, this book concentrates on mental and emotional strain rather than on physical stressors and responses. Stressors would include a wide variety of external stimuli, such as job stressors, personal or social stimuli, or personal performance expectations. It is important to recognize that all of these are strongly individual and may even be self-imposed. The stressfulness of an environment must encompass all the stressors that can contribute to the wear and tear on the body, mind, and health of the individual by affecting the musculoskeletal system, the cardiovascular system, the

1

respiratory system, and other body systems. The mechanisms may involve the endocrine system, the metabolic system, the cardiovascular system, the immune system, and the gastrointestinal system, among others.

In our practice we measure the impact of mental stress in a clinical setting by determining the response (in terms of the quality and quantity of reactivity) of a given system to a controlled (standardized) input stressor. Thus, standardized low-challenge stressors can be designed to elucidate the effects, if any, on any of the above systems, and measurements can be obtained in a reasonably objective fashion. The real question then is how do these laboratory measurements relate to and predict reactivity in the real world, in real-time settings? In my view, this is the name of the game in contemporary research and clinical medicine. Naturally, pencil and paper tests, interview, and other techniques are supplementary in making reasonable clinical predictions.

In addition, it is important to expand our understanding of reactivity beyond the hemodynamic or physiologic reactivity that relates to the cardiovascular system. For example, lipid metabolism also responds to stressors. In a study of CPAs, Friedman and Rosenman[1] noted a significant rise in serum cholesterol levels of as much as a hundred milligrams percent between January 1 and April 15, even without significant changes in diet. This suggests what could be termed "metabolic reactivity" to stressors by accountants during tax season.

Endocrine reactivity can also be demonstrated, for example, by measuring noradrenalin and adrenaline levels during time-reaction tests. By using "wet Holter monitoring" (automatic blood sampling of ambulatory subjects) to determine endocrine levels during various activities, Dimsdale[2] beautifully demonstrated the impact of environmental stress, finding extremely low levels at rest and maximum levels during public speaking or dental procedures.

Another example of environmental stress effects can be found in the work of Kaplan et al.[3] which demonstrated a greater incidence of lesions in the arterial intima of animals in very stressful environments compared to those in low-stress environments. In a subsequent study,[4] they compared high and low reactors using heart rate as the end point. They found a twofold difference in the degree of atherosclerosis in high reactors as compared to low reactors. Although such correlation does not prove cause and effect, it suggests the importance and the impact of the stressor environment on the process of atherosclerosis.

External chemical factors also influence reactivity. For example,

MacDougall et al.[5] have demonstrated that cigarette smokers show greater hemodynamic reactivity than non-smokers. Indeed, the effects of emotional stressors and smoking are additive. Further studies are needed with regard to the impact of smoking, salt, caffeine, exercise, and other factors on reactivity. Interactions as well as the factors themselves must be considered.

Coronary-prone behavior has been much discussed over the past five years. One form of behavior alleged to be "coronary prone" is the well-known type A behavior. Some studies have reported that the risk of coronary heart disease for type A individuals is double that of type Bs. Other studies, however, have failed to find any significant correlation. Where does the truth lie?

Some investigations are now focusing on various components of type A. Free-floating hostility and anger inward both show some promise as prognostic factors. For instance, there is some evidence that individuals who feel hostile but cannot express it, are more apt to be reactive. Again Kaplan et al.[6] have demonstrated in a heart-rate study with animals that high-reactive animals are far more aggressive than normal or low-reactive animals. Human studies from Williams et al.[7] demonstrated that the female who has the lowest hostility and the least type A behavior has the lowest incidence and least severity of coronary artery disease by angiography (in terms of percent occlusion). The highest level, by contrast, is in the male type A with the greatest hostility. In these studies, the relationship is reported to be linear.

Environmental considerations such as social support, work demands, life change events, and neighborhood security appear to have a relationship to coronary heart disease. A common factor seems to be the need to feel in control of one's life. For example, Karasek et al.[8] found that job decision latitude is more important than job demand. High job demand is not necessarily stressful if there is considerable decision latitude. However, as latitude decreases and the sense of being in control diminishes, there is considerable increase in the incidence of coronary heart disease. Thus, work conditions such as long hours, heavy responsibilities, or time constraints should be viewed in context with decision-making latitude.

With regard to intervention, clearly identification of the problem is only 20% of the issue; helping individuals to change and motivating them to do so constitutes the other 80%. It is necessary to alter either the stressful environment or the individual's stress response or both. On an individual basis it is often almost impossible to change the environment as we tend to be locked into relatively rigid environmental patterns. We are more successful in changing our perception of events or stressors and the body's physiological response. These changes can sometimes be accomplished pharmacologically; for example, beta blockers have been successful in reducing the anxiety associated with public speaking. Nonpharmacologic efforts such as relaxation and biofeedback techniques are proving increasingly valuable and effective for self-regulation. Surwit at Duke University[9] showed that individuals who learned these techniques and implemented them at times of perceived stress and known elevations of blood pressure could blunt inappropriate reactivity ("hot reacting"). At the end of treatment the relative magnitude of systolic and diastolic elevations was significantly reduced. Other behavioral therapies have also been of value.

Unquestionably, the brain reigns supreme in this rapidly unfolding field. Only recently it has been discovered that the brain produces as many as 10,000 neuropeptide hormones that regulate much of the neurochemical and neurophysiologic outflow to the body. Skinner[10] has shown that the pathways from the frontal lobes govern critical steps that affect lipid metabolism, ventricular fibrillatory threshold, hypertension, and other cardiovascular phenomena.

Thus, over the past five years, investigations into the role of lifestyle, behavior, and stress in cardiovascular disease, have achieved remarkable and significant progress in uncovering mechanisms, developing objective techniques for assessment, and implementing new pharmacological and nonpharmacological management techniques, all of which enhance our clinical understanding and success in dealing with cardiovascular disease. There is still a need to investigate the multiple factors and physiological hierarchies that contribute to stress-linked illnesses: from the basic cellular to the biochemical to the metabolic to the physiologic to the psychologic and sociocultural levels. Considering the remarkable progress that has been made within the last five years, one can be optimistic about future develoments.

This text is designed for health professionals who seek a broad practical understanding of this field. It is not oriented toward theoretical and basic science. The latest "state-of-the-art" knowledge of the mechanisms, assessment techniques and management systems are discussed primarily as they apply to clinical medicine today.

For certain chapters, where appropriate and where special areas are addressed, additional resource experts have been added. Those selected have made major contributions to our knowledge and, importantly, have translated their findings into practical clinical terms.

I hope this text will enrich both your personal and professional lives.

Robert S. Eliot, M.D.

References

1. Friedman M, Rosenman RH, Carroll V. Changes in the serum cholesterol and blood clotting time in men subjected to cyclic variation of occupational stress. Circulation 17:852–861, 1958.
2. Dimsdale JE. Wet Holter monitoring: Techniques for studying plasma responses to stress in ambulatory subjects. In: Dembroski TM, Schmidt TH, Blumchen G (eds). Biobehavioral Bases of Coronary Heart Disease. Karger, Basel, 1983, pp 175–184.
3. Kaplan JR, Manuck SB, Clarkson TB, et al. Social stress and atherosclerosis in normocholesterolemic monkeys. Science 220:733–735, 1983.
4. Kaplan JR, Manuck SB. Stress-induced heart rate reactivity and atherosclerosis in monkeys. Psychosom Med 43:189, 1981.
5. MacDougall JM, Dembroski TM, Slaats S, et al. Selective cardiovascular effects of stress and cigarette smoking. J Hum Stress 9(3):13–21, 1983.
6. Kaplan JR, Manuck SB, Clarkson TB: Psychosocial stress and atherosclerosis in cynomolgus macaques. In: Beamish RE, Singal PK, Dhalla NS, (eds). Stress and Heart Disease, Martinus Nijhoff Publishing, Boston, 1985, pp 262–276.
7. Williams RB, Haney TL, Lee KL, et al. Type A behavior, hostility, and coronary atherosclerosis. Psychosom Med 42:539–549, 1980.
8. Karasek R, Baker D, Marxer F, et al. Job decision latitude, job demands, and cardiovascular disease: a prospective study of Swedish men. Am J Pub Health 71:694–705, 1981.
9. Surwit RS, Williams RB Jr, Shapiro D. Behavioral Approaches to Cardiovascular Disease. Academic Press, New York, 1982.
10. Skinner JE: Psychosocial stress and sudden cardiac death: brain mechanisms. In: Beamish RE, Singal PK, Dhalla NS (eds). Stress and Heart Disease, Martinus Nijhoff Publishing, Boston, 1985, pp 44–59.

Mechanisms Linking Stress to Cardiovascular Damage

Chapter 1

Risk Factors

Robert S. Eliot

Introduction

There are many instances of persons dying suddenly after an emotional upset. In the past two decades, evidence documenting the profound effects of stress on human and animal physiology has confirmed the link between emotions and illness or death.

More and more studies implicate psychosocial conflict, emotions, and behavioral patterns in the pathogenesis of coronary heart disease, sudden death, cardiac arrhythmias, and systemic hypertension. Interest in the roles played by stress and the central nervous system in these disorders has been heightened by the observation that the traditional risk factors fail to account for half the cases of clinical coronary heart disease.[1]

Stress remains to be well defined. In the context of this discussion, stress is considered to be the body's response to real or imagined events perceived as requiring some adaptive response and/or producing strain. This often results from a mismatch between what a person would like to have happen and what the world delivers.

Utility of Risk Factors

As Kannel and Schatzkin[2] point out, the "risk factor" term has three connotations: (1) a statistical correlate of coronary heart disease

From: Eliot, RS: *Stress and the Heart: Mechanisms, Measurements and Management.* Mount Kisco, NY, Futura Publishing Company, Inc., © 1988.

(CHD), (2) a cause of CHD, and (3) a characteristic that predisposes to CHD. Less than 50% of CHD cases are accounted for by the recognized risk factors of elevated cholesterol, hypertension, cigarette smoking, diabetes mellitus, family history, and obesity. That is, half of CHD cases occur among people not significantly different from those free of disease. The other half occur among the 20% of the population who have significantly higher levels or numbers of risk factors. However, the incidence even in people with 5 factors is only 63% over 8 years[3] and, therefore, absolute causation has been, and remains, hard to prove. Rather, risk factor analyses are useful in predicting susceptibility to CHD and for indicating areas for health improvement in high-risk individuals.[4]

It is difficult to separate the roles of behavior and environment from the accepted risk factors. Each risk factor is a composite of genetic, environmental, and behavioral components, and the interactions that generate or sustain them can be very complex.

Cholesterol

Cholesterol may be the most important of the risk factors. The higher levels of the low density lipoproteins (LDL) increase atherogenic risk. The higher levels of high density lipoprotein (HDL) decrease atherogenic risk. Both animal and human studies have shown strong association between CHD and serum total cholesterol level. Furthermore, it appears that only the LDL component is atherogenic and that certain fractions of the HDL component are actually protective.[5,6] However, epidemiologic studies show excess mortality at both extremes of serum cholesterol distribution: deaths at the lower extremes from cancer and at the higher levels from CHD. The lowest rates of CHD are associated with average population cholesterol values of 140 to 180 mg/dl.[7]

The relation of diet to serum cholesterol levels is still not completely clear. While dietary fat intake appears to be statistically significant, dietary cholesterol is not all absorbed and most cholesterol found in the serum is actually manufactured in the liver; this suggests that factors other than diet are involved.

It has been demonstrated that some normal people can maintain an acceptable cholesterol level even on a diet of high cholesterol foods,[8] while susceptible individuals increase their blood cholesterol under stress even on a diet of low cholesterol foods. For instance, accountants studied by Friedman et al.[9] had demonstrated the highest serum cholesterol levels during periods of severe occupational and emotional stress and the lowest levels during periods of minimal stress, without changes in dietary fat intake.

Empirical evidence seems to support the hypothesis that, generally, the lower the saturated fats and cholesterol in the diet of a population, the lower the incidence of CHD. Modifications in diet to reduce the fats and cholesterol, as in the Oslo Study Group,[10] were also associated with lower mortality rates than in control groups.

Hypertension

Hypertension affects approximately forty million Americans. Yet it cannot be traced to an identifiable cause in more than 90% of the cases.[11] Much of the reduction in coronary mortality over the past decades has been attributed to greater efforts and increased effectiveness in antihypertensive therapy. While the necessity for treatment of mild hypertension may be controversial, there is considerable evidence that the risk of cardiovascular disease and death increase with increasing blood pressure and that proper treatment significantly prolongs life.[12]

Although in our society, blood pressure has a general tendency to rise with age, the increase is associated with no less risk for older persons than for younger individuals. The systolic blood pressure increases more with age than the diastolic and, in elderly people, overall mortality seems to correlate with the systolic pressure, independent of the diastolic. The pathological result of hypertension in the elderly is more apt to be stroke and less likely to be occlusive peripheral arterial disease.

Many laymen have the misconception that an inner feeling of nervous tension indicates hypertension, but, while this is not the case, there are strong suggestions that psychosocial and behavioral factors do have a part in the pathogenesis of hypertension. Henry and Ely,[13] for instance, found that fixed hypertension and myocardial hypertrophy, progressive arteriosclerosis, myocardial fibrosis, and renal failure can be induced in mice that have been raised in isolation, simply by putting them into a cage with other mice, thus subjecting them to social interaction. Other psychosocial factors leading to hypertension are described in Chapter 3 The Role of Environment.

Cigarette Smoking

Clearly cigarette smoking is the least controversial of the CHD risk factors. Smoking behavior often starts as the result of peer pressure and then continues as a coping mode. While the overall extent of smoking has declined markedly in recent years, there has been less of a decline among blacks and women than among white males. In some cases, cessation of smoking is accompanied by withdrawal symptoms like those from addictive drugs, but in others no such symptoms occur. In general, the longer the habit has been established and the more cigarettes smoked per day, the harder it is to stop. The cardiovascular risk is more related to the number smoked per day than to duration.[14]

The prevalence of CHD doubles in cigarette smokers versus nonsmokers and the statistical relation of cigarette smoking to CHD is particularly compelling as a potentiator in the presence of other risk factors such as high serum cholesterol.[15] For those who quit smoking, the risk of myocardial infarction (MI) drops and over many years the risk approaches that of individuals who had never smoked.[15] In my view, this probably results partly from the adoption of improved coping mechanisms.

Various explanations have been offered for the pathologic effects of cigarette smoking. Since cigarette smoking releases a number of noxious components (nicotine and carbon monoxide being the major ones), the mechanisms may well be complex and interactive. Carbon monoxide, of course, reduces the oxygen available, and nicotine stimulates catecholamine release which increases oxygen demand and has profound effects on the cardiovascular system and the central nervous system (CNS).[16]

Obesity

Obesity can be the result of eating habits that have been culturally ingrained and/or be a coping behavior. There is also a strong genetic factor.

Moderate obesity unaccompanied by other risk factors seems to convey little risk of cardiovascular disease. However, gross obesity (more than 20% above the top of the recommended weight range of the 1983 Metropolitan Life Insurance Company table) is often associated with hypertension[17] and increased cholesterol.[18] When fat cells are greatly distended, disorders of glucose metabolism are common and insulin production may increase.[19] Type II diabetes, which is found more frequently among obese women than those of normal weight, often can be better controlled or may even disappear with weight loss. However, even when diabetes is under control, diabetics are more susceptible to cardiovascular illness.

Obesity is related particularly to angina pectoris and sudden death. The incidence of sudden death increases with the degree of overweight for men. In women the triad of obesity, diabetes, and low HDL cholesterol carries an especially high risk of CHD.[20] Abdominal fat appears to convey a greater risk than hip and thigh fat. In men a waist/hip ratio above 1.0 is a risk factor for ischemic heart disease, stroke, diabetes mellitus, and death; in women the risks rise with a ratio above 0.8.[21]

Cardiac output in obese persons is elevated because of the increased tissue demands and blood volumes. This results in increased right heart filling pressures roughly proportional to the degree of obesity.[19]

Diabetes Mellitus

The risk of CHD is doubled for diabetic men and tripled for diabetic women. Although diabetics also tend to have other risk factors, especially high blood pressure and obesity, the excess risk cannot be entirely attributed to these associated factors.[2] Framingham studies and others show the relative impact of diabetes is greatest for occlusive peripheral arterial disease, but CHD occurs more frequently.

While stress is not strongly implicated in the pathogenesis of diabetes, it is known to disrupt diabetic control, perhaps because of increased cortisol and catecholamines.

Family History

The Framingham study showed familial vulnerability to CHD independent of other known risk factors. Persons whose first-degree relatives (parents, siblings, children) have had premature CHD have a risk two to five times that of persons with a negative family history. Family history is less conclusively implicated in stroke. A familial tendency in hypertension has been documented. The hereditary susceptibility to hypertension may, however, be manifested only in combination with other factors such as sustained stress or high salt load.[22] The frequent concordance on cholesterol levels observed in spouses in the Framingham study suggests that environmental effects may be as important as genetic ones in familial tendencies.

In a nine-year study of 4014 men and women in Rancho Bernardo, California, Barrett-Conner and Khaw[23] used the Cox proportional hazards model to assess cardiovascular risks. They reported a significant excess risk of cardiovascular death associated with positive family history only in men less than 60 years of age. Family history was not predictive for men over 60 or for women in any age group.

Sedentary Behavior

Regular physical activity, whether work or leisure seems, in some instances, to offer protection from the complications of CHD. However, vigorous exercise, such as jogging and logging, has also been associated with numerous deaths. Apparently the level required to confer benefit depends on an interrelationship with other factors. Keys[24] found inconsistencies in the results of studies in different nations and noted that: "in regard to mortality and physical activity, it is possible to select among cohorts so as to support whatever predilection is espoused."

An ongoing study of Harvard alumni[25] showed that after 12 to 16 years of follow-up, those who regularly expended at least 2,000 calories per week in physical activity had lower than average mortality, and the greater the activity level the lower the mortality rate. Whether this study isolates physical activity as a clear benefit or as an indicator of pre-existing good health remains to be demonstrated. In addition, one must also consider that the discipline needed to be regularly active over 12 years will also be directed at other risk factors and lifestyle considerations. Again, it is nearly impossible in any human study to isolate all other interacting factors from a single solitary targeted risk factor. Keys' remarks quoted above and Irvine Page's theory of mosaic risk patterns[26] remain cogent and timely.

References

1. Gordon T, Kannel WB. Multiple risk functions for predicting coronary heart disease: the concept, accuracy, and application. Am Heart J 103:1031–1039, 1982.
2. Kannel WB, Schatzkin A. Risk factor analysis. Progress in Cardiovascular Diseases 26(4):309–332, 1983.
3. McGee D. The probability of developing certain cardiovascular diseases in 8 years at specified values of some characteristics. Section 28 In: Kannel WB, Gordon T (eds). The Framingham Study. National Heart Lung Inst. National Institutes of Health, Pub. No. (NIH) 74-618, Washington, DC, Government Printing Office, 1973.

4. Kannel WB, McGee D, Gordon T. A general cardiovascular risk profile: The Framingham Study. Am J Cardiol 38:46–51, 1976.
5. Castelli WP, Doyle JT, Gordon T, et al. HDL cholesterol and other lipids in coronary heart disease. The cooperative lipoprotein phenotyping study. Circulation 55:767, 1977.
6. Carew TE, Koschinsky T, Hayes SB, et al. A mechanism by which high-density lipoprotein may slow the atherogenic process. Lancet 1:1315, 1976.
7. Atherosclerosis Study Group (Kannel WB, Chairman). Optimal resources for primary prevention of atherosclerotic diseases. Circulation 70:155A–205A, 1984.
8. Kannel WB, Gordon T, (eds). The Framingham Study: an epidemiological investigation of cardiovascular disease. Section 24. Diet and the regulation of serum cholesterol. Washington, DC, Government Printing Office, 1970.
9. Friedman M, Rosenman RH, Carroll V. Changes in the serum cholesterol and blood clotting time in men subjected to cyclic variation of occupational stress. Circulation 17:852, 1958.
10. Hjermann I, Velve Byre K, Leren P. Effect of diet and smoking on the incidence of coronary heart disease: Report from the Oslo Study Group of a randomised trial in healthy men. Lancet 2:1303, 1981.
11. Folkow B. Physiological aspects of primary hypertension. Physiol Rev 62:347–504, 1982.
12. The Joint National Committee on Detection, Evaluation, and Treatment of High Blood Pressure. The 1984 report of the Joint National Committee on Detection, Evaluation, and Treatment of High Blood Pressure. Arch Intern Med 144:1045–1057, 1984.
13. Henry JP, Ely DL. Physiology of emotional stress. Specific responses. J SC Med Assoc 75:501, 1979.
14. Kannel WB: Update on the role of cigarette smoking in coronary artery disease. Am Heart J 101:319–328, 1981.
15. Kannel WB, Stokes J III. The epidemiology of coronary artery disease. In: Cohn PF (ed). Diagnosis and Therapy of Coronary Artery Disease. Martinus Nijhoff Publishing, Boston 1985, pp 63–88.
16. Klein LW, Pichard AD, Holt J, et al. Effects of chronic tobacco smoking on the coronary circulation. J Am Coll Cardiol 1:421–426, 1983.
17. Dustan HP. Obesity and hypertension. Ann Intern Med 103 (6, suppl., Part 2):1047–1049, 1985.
18. Bray GA. Complications of obesity. Ann Intern Med 103 (6, suppl., Part 2):1052–1062, 1985.
19. Arik TH, Desser KB, Benchimol A. Obesity and heart disease. Ariz Med 42(1):12–13, 1985.
20. Kannel WB, Gordon T, Castelli WP: Obesity, lipids and glucose intolerance: the Framingham study. Am J Clin Nutr 32:1238, 1979.
21. Bjorntorp P. Regional patterns of fat distribution. Ann Int Med 103 (6 pt 2):994–995, 1985.
22. Falkner B, Onesti G, Angelakos E. Effect of salt loading on the cardiovascular response to stress in adolescents. Proceedings/Interamerican Society Supp II Hypertension 3:II-195–II-199, 1981.

23. Barrett-Conner E, Khaw K. Family history of heart attack as an independent predictor of death due to cardiovascular disease. Circulation 69:1065–1069, 1984.
24. Keys A. Ten-year mortality in the seven countries study. In: Medical Aspects of Mortality Statistics, Bostrom H, Ljungstedt N (ed). The Skandia Group, Almqvist & Wiksell International, Stockholm, 1981.
25. Paffenbarger RS, Hyde RT, Wing AL, et al. Physical activity, all-cause mortality, and longevity of college alumni. N Engl J Med 314:605–613, 1986.
26. Page IH. Pathogenesis of arterial hypertension. JAMA 140:451–457, 1949.

Chapter 2

Coronary-Prone Behavior

Robert S. Eliot

Even though Sir William Osler, as early as 1910 described an apparent relationship between arteriosclerosis and a high-pressure life,[1] the issue of psychosocial factors in coronary heart disease did not receive much attention until Friedman and Rosenman[2] described and popularized the term "type A" almost a half century later. The fully developed type A behavior pattern connotes speed, impatience, hostility, competitive drive, and a sense of an effort-oriented person caught up in a joyless struggle. The diagnosis is made classically using a structured interview with the subjects' responses taped and graded for mannerisms and verbal styles of loud, explosive, rapid, and accelerated speech, hostility, etc.: a total of 22 affects. It has been validated primarily in the demographically restricted group of middle- and upper-class employed American men over 39 years of age.

Changes in the constellation of characteristics, the way the interview is conducted, substitution of written tests, and problems of reproducibility among interviewers have cast doubts on the relevance and comparability of studies. For example, one version of the structured interview used in MRFIT[3] classified 75% of subjects as type A. In the original WCGS study[4], only 50% of subjects were classified as type A.

Dimsdale[5] has thoroughly reviewed the controversies regarding type A behavior. He suggests that the inconsistency between early studies that found type A predictive of coronary heart disease and later studies such as MRFIT that found it unrelated may be caused by a change in the type A classification (the structured interview is difficult

From: Eliot, RS: *Stress and the Heart: Mechanisms, Measurements and Management.* Mount Kisco, NY, Futura Publishing Company, Inc., © 1988.

to standardize) or in the populations studied. He points out that recent reviews of the Framingham study found type A behavior associated with risk in men employed in white-collar jobs but not in men in blue-collar jobs. The overall drop in CHD mortality noted in the last decade has been largely among middle-class males; now blue-collar workers are the group most at risk. It may be that only certain elements of the type A pattern are pertinent in determining risk, or it may be that only a select population is at risk from the type A pattern. Dimsdale believes that "if type A behavior is to survive as a risk factor, this original simplicity must be replaced by a more complex description of the behaviors and the populations at risk for such behaviors."

It is important to make a distinction, then, between type A behavior and the ill-defined but constantly evolving concept of coronary-prone behavior. Individuals manifesting type A behavior may survive unscathed into old age, attending the funerals of their younger type B counterparts. The association remains incomplete although it appears that certain components of type A behavior may be predictive of CHD.

Glass[6] observed that depression in the type A personality was significantly related to CHD. His findings are in accord with a study by Thomas et al.[7] of physicians with myocardial infarcts (MI) who readily became depressed even as students. It also supports the conclusions of Bruhn et al.[8] that the coronary-prone individual is an effort-oriented person whose achievements give him little satisfaction.

A study by Dembroski et al.[9] of coronary and noncoronary patients, illustrates the discrepancy between coronary-prone behavior and type A. During a structured interview and an American history quiz, they noted an increase in systolic blood pressure during the history quiz in type B coronary patients but not in type B controls. Indeed, the greatest increment of blood pressure change in either type A or B groups was evoked in type B MI patients during the American history quiz.

Alexander[10] characterized the hypertensive personality as one who inhibits rage and anger and turns them inward. Esler et al.[11] have reported that psychometric testing of patients with high renin hypertension revealed suppressed hostility linked to increased sympathetic activity. The individuals were described as withdrawn, not easily communicative, and tending to avoid confrontation with people when rage would be justified. Manuck et al.[12] also noted a difference in personality between high renin hypertensives and other hypertensives. They suggested that high renin personality may reflect a general lack of aggressiveness either as a method of coping or as the result of social deficiencies.

Such observations suggest that coronary proneness is not congruent with any one type of behavior or personality but results from the integration of these aspects with individual perceptions and physiological tendencies.

In our experience the most consistent factors preceding CHD seem to be associated with key personal struggles leading to the perception of defeat: a sense of loss of control, loss of identity, and/or loss of self-esteem. This feeling may be precipitated by loss of one's job as we noted in the Kennedy aerospace engineers[13]; by the death of a spouse; by divorce; by business failures; by changes in acculturation as in immigration to a new country or from rural to urban areas or the move by an elderly person from home to a nursing facility.

Among women, the highest incidence of CHD in the Framingham study[14] occurred among clerical workers who had an oppressive boss, were married to a blue-collar worker, and had several children. Consumption of one or more packs of cigarettes per day, recent loss of a "significant other," and a history of psychiatric illness, such as depression, also increased the risks for women.

However, all the aspects of coronary-prone behavior are subject to the mitigating and mutating effects of genetic predisposition, cultural cohesion, coping strategies, and dietary habits. Even cigarette smoking, which has such consistently dire consequences in the United States, does not necessarily correlate with increased coronary heart disease in other locales, such as Japan.[15]

Clearly the perception and response to a variety of environmental challenges, the existence of support systems, and the availability of such factors as coping style and hardiness, for example, help to swing the balance and to distinguish those who survive and flourish versus those who succumb. An overview of environmental influences will now serve to enhance the reader's understanding of the clinical importance of these factors.

References

1. Osler W. The Lumleian lectures on angina pectoris. Lancet 1:839–844, 1910.
2. Friedman M, Rosenman RH. Association of specific overt behavior pattern with increases in blood cholesterol, blood clotting time, incidence of arcus senilis and clinical coronary heart disease. JAMA 169:1286–1296, 1959.
3. MRFIT Research Group. Risk factor changes and mortality results. JAMA 248:1465–1477, 1982.

4. Rosenman RH, et al. Coronary heart disease in the Western Collaborative Group Study: final follow-up experience of $8\frac{1}{2}$ years. JAMA 233:872–877, 1975.

5. Dimsdale JE. Controversies regarding type A behavior and coronary heart disease. Cardiol Clin 3(2):259–267, 1985.

6. Glass DC: Behavior Patterns, Stress and Coronary Disease. Lawrence Erlbaum, Hillsdale, NJ, 1977.

7. Thomas CB, Ross DC, Duszynski KR. Youthful hypercholesterolemia: its associated characteristics and role in premature myocardial infarction. Johns Hopkins Med J 136:193–208, 1975.

8. Bruhn JG, Paredes A, Adsett CA, et al. Psychological predictors of sudden death in myocardial infarction. Journal of Psychosomatic Research 18:187–191, 1974.

9. Dembroski TM, MacDougall JM, Lushene R. Interpersonal interaction and cardiovascular response in type A subjects and coronary patients. J of Hum Stress 5:28–36, 1979.

10. Alexander FW. Psychosomatic Medicine: Its Principles and Applications. W. W. Norton and Co., New York, 1950.

11. Esler M, Julius S, Zweifler A, et al. Mild high-renin essential hypertension: neurogenic human hypertension? NEJM 296:405–11, 1977.

12. Manuck SB, Garland FN. Coronary-prone behavior pattern, task incentive and cardiovascular response. Psychophysiology 16:136, 1979.

13. Eliot RS, (ed). Stress and the Heart. Futura Publishing Co., Mount Kisco, N.Y. 1974.

14. Haynes SG, Feinleib M. Women, work and coronary heart disease: prospective findings from the Framingham heart study. Am J of Public Health 70:133–141, 1980.

15. Keys A, (ed). Coronary heart disease in seven countries. Circulation Suppl. 1 42:I-1–I-211, 1970.

Chapter 3

The Role of Environment

Robert S. Eliot
W. Thomas Boyce

Although health practitioners now recognize the impact of behavior on disease, we tend to overlook the importance of the environment in which that behavior takes place. The interaction between the individual and the environment is important, because stress is largely a product of the environmental context.

Epidemiologists who are disease oriented see the environment as the source of vectors or agents, such as viruses, animals, physicochemical agents, or water supplies. The role of environment is quite different in noninfectious diseases. The determination of psychosocial factors, such as mobility, is far more pertinent. Social status, interactions with other people, and changes in such social elements impact on health. When people change jobs, change residences, or make other major life changes, the risk of heart disease goes up two to three times, independent of such factors as age, sex, race, cigarette smoking, cholesterol, blood pressure history, physical activity, and obesity.

Harburg and colleagues[1] have shown that blacks living in areas of Detroit with low ecologic stress had less hypertension than their counterparts living in high stress areas. Gampel et al[2] noted a lower incidence of hypertension among Zulus in rural areas than among those who moved to the cities; the urban Zulus who were hypertensive tended to be those who clung to traditional cultural practices and seemed unable to adapt to the demands of urban living.

From: Eliot, RS: *Stress and the Heart: Mechanisms, Measurements and Management.* Mount Kisco, NY, Futura Publishing Company, Inc., © 1988.

Social Support

Syme's group studied a Japanese population of 17,000 that migrated from the southwestern prefectures of Japan to Oahu and the Bay Area of California.[3-5] They found a marked increase in coronary heart disease—up to fivefold among Japanese that migrated to California and a lesser increase in those who migrated to Hawaii. However, among the Japanese migrants in California he noted a group who had almost the same low incidence of coronary disease as those who remained in Japan, suggesting that mobility per se was not a major risk factor for the migrants.

In view of the highly urbanized industrialized society in Japan, with marked air pollution, excessive smoking, and crowding, one might logically assume that genetic factors would explain why the Japanese have the lowest incidence of heart disease in the world. However, the increased incidence among most Japanese-Americans proved that this was not the case. Another reasonable hypothesis focusing on diet changes—from rice and fish to the "Big Mac" hamburger (that is, from complex carbohydrate to beef tallow)—also did not explain the differences among the migrants. Nor could the fivefold increase be explained by their serum cholesterol levels, blood pressure, or smoking habits.

Michael Marmot in cooperation with Dr. Syme compared two subpopulations of the Japanese migrants with markedly different rates of coronary heart disease.[6] The group with the higher rate had become acculturated and had adopted "Western ways." Those with low incidence of heart disease had been raised in a Japanese neighborhood, with Japanese friends, Japanese language, and other cultural habits and had maintained a strong interest in Japanese customs and beliefs as adults. The research team concluded that the main difference between the groups was the degree of social support. Clearly, the Japanese have a strong sense of community, and various social support networks that are in place from earliest childhood are maintained throughout life. To many Japanese, this is the most profound difference between living in Japan and living in the United States.

To verify the importance of social support networks, Berkman and Syme[7] surveyed a more general population of about 7,000 in Alameda County of California. They were evaluated on the basis of such criteria as whether they were married, belonged to clubs, and/or attended a church or synagogue. Then researchers recorded the mortality over the next nine years for the different groupings. Those with fewer connections at the beginning of the study had a much higher mortality rate. Even when taking account of such factors as age, race, cigarette smoking, serum cholesterol, blood pressure, family history, physical activity, obesity, socioeconomic status, and self-reported health status, the risks for those with few social associations were two to three times those having the greatest number of connections.

Curiously, the data were for all forms of death, not just heart disease alone. Somehow, the absence of an appropriate support network compromises the body's defense system in general, increasing the individual's vulnerability (or the presence of supports offers added protection). Thus it appears that the defense system may be affected by a variety of factors including social relationships, genetic predisposition, nutritional status, and previous exposure. Indeed, vulnerability in this sense may not predict the cause of death but rather the risk of dying.

The protective effects of social support help to explain two questions raised by morbidity data: (1) Why do the recognized risk factors, such as cigarette smoking, high blood pressure, and elevated serum cholesterol relate so imperfectly with disease incidence and outcome? It may be that 90% of people are protected from the adverse effects of these factors. (2) Why are certain risk factors related not just to one disease but to a variety of diseases. For instance, with regard to type A behavior, it may be that type A individuals are too busy to maintain relationships with others; maintaining intimate ties with others takes energy and is often viewed as nonproductive, especially by driven type A individuals.

In Syme's view, life-changes are important primarily when they disrupt relationships, such as would happen with job changes, residential moves, divorce, or the loss of loved ones. Even the difference between male and female risks in CHD may be related to social support. As Syme has reported, men seem to have few intimate ties, with the exception of their wives or another woman, while women have many more close relationships.

Indeed when Syme reviewed his impressions of the MRFIT program, he recalled that at the start, many individuals in the intervention group told him that they "really didn't have time to participate in the groups." They requested that they be given the material so they could do the exercises at home. The participants were told that the agreement required them to come for ten sessions over a ten-week period and that they couldn't just work at home. It was thus a real surprise after the tenth session when the participants asked for additional sessions. When informed that only ten sessions were included in the protocol, they even suggested meeting in their own homes. Apparently these individuals had developed a meaningful relationship with the group and wished to maintain it.

By contrast, in Japan close relationships are taken for granted. There, people are born into a group setting, they go through school together, take a job together, go through their entire work experience as a group, and even picnic and vacation together. They continue to maintain close contacts with relatives and friends in the place where they grew up. If their jobs have taken them elsewhere, they still generally return to their original home when they retire. How many of us could return to our home town and find people we knew when we were growing up? How many of us have kept contact with the same friends from childhood throughout life?

The effect of social contact can even be seen in animal studies. Nerem et al.[8] found that rabbits that were fondled and petted while on a high cholesterol diet had a markedly lower rate of atherogenesis than a matched group that was not fondled.

A support system is needed by all of us who have to deal with personal problems. For example, if you need money, is there someone you can turn to for a loan? If you need a ride is there someone who will provide it? If you need help with household chores, is there someone you can ask? If a dear one dies, is there someone nearby to offer comfort? It should be emphasized that very often health relates more to the perceived level of support than to the actual level of support that is available.

Dr. Therese Seeman[9] (a student of Syme) examined the social supports of a group of people undergoing coronary angiography. She asked how many friends they had, whether they felt isolated, whether friends were important, whether they were satisfied with the people they knew, and whether they helped each other or felt they could rely on friends for help when needed. She found that functional support but not emotional support correlated with less coronary artery disease.

An interesting study[10] was conducted in children who were placed in the Headstart Program. By the fourth grade, they no longer performed better in school than those who had not been in the program. However, later they demonstrated lower incidences of teenage pregnancy, school dropout, minor violations of the law, criminal arrests, unemployment, and smoking, and had a higher rate of college attendance. Several studies of educational strategies show similar results. Even at that early age, establishment of identity, self-esteem and social support provides lasting benefits.

The impact of social support and the cultural climate are evident in various other studies. The cultural milieu often defines such factors as diet, attitude to older people, and social interaction. In studies of the Italian-American town of Roseto,[11] the incidence of heart attacks was low (half that of neighboring towns) as long as the community was committed to the Old World values, which included deep religious convictions, respect for the elderly, subordination of women to men, and conformity to Italian traditions. The difference could not be explained by differences in any of the usually accepted risk factors. Over a twenty-year period, as the community became more Americanized and less cohesive, the incidence of coronary heart disease rose to approximate that of the surrounding towns.

The effect of diet is notable in the contrasting incidence of coronary diseases in the Mediterranean versus the Scandinavian countries where the incidence is very high. The diet characteristic of the Mediterranean countries, such as Italy and Greece, emphasizes the use of olive oil (a monounsaturated fat), rice, and other carbohydrates, and poultry and fish rather than red meat. Wine is a common accompaniment of food. In the Scandinavian countries, dairy products and red meat are important elements, while carbohydrates and vegetables have a lesser role in the diet. When a group of Finns were put on a Mediterranean-style diet their total serum cholesterol decreased significantly.[12]

Social Class

Socioeconomic factors have been correlated with health. The lower the socioeconomic status the higher the rates of virtually every disease. The reasons for this difference are not clearly understood. Hypotheses include poor nutrition, poor medical care, heavy infectious burden, etc., but these variables do not entirely account for the differences. There is a gradient of decreasing rates from the lowest socioeconomic to the highest socioeconomic levels. Age, sex, availability of medical care, alcohol intake, physical activity, and the cardiovascular risk factors have all failed to explain this.

The Oslo study[13] noted that coronary risk was related to social class. The authors defined five social classes by gross income and years of education. Coronary risk factors, especially cigarette smoking and elevated serum cholesterol, were higher among the lower classes such that the risk in class 5 (lowest education and income) was about 2.5 times that of class 1 (highest education and income). Mortality from

CHD, as well as from other causes, such as cancer and accidents, followed this same pattern. In social class 3, income and educational levels were mixed: it included some financially successful men with little education and some highly educated men with low income. Interestingly, the highly educated men of low income (whom they dubbed "underachievers") had only two thirds of the coronary risk of the successful men of less education.

In the Whitehall study of London civil servants,[14] the mortality of those in the lowest pay grade was four times that of the highest grade. However, difference in risk factors accounted for less than half of the variation.

Some of the differences between social classes may be the result of environmental factors in the work or residential areas. Climate, urban/rural locale, noise, even architecture can influence health. Extremes of temperature are stressful to persons not acclimated or properly dressed for it.

In the Alameda County study, a poverty area was compared with a more affluent area. Incidence of hypertension was 50% higher in the poverty area regardless of considerations of social interaction, medical care, smoking, and other accepted risk factors. However, among a group of more affluent people living in the area, the pattern of hypertension reflected that of the poverty area as a whole rather than that of the similar income group in the affluent area. Interviews with the individuals revealed fears of robbery and violence. It was then noted that the distribution of hypertension within the community correlated with the concentration of police and fire department calls.

Architecture

Architectural design and city layout influence behavior and thus affect health. For instance, they tend to encourage sedentary behavior rather than healthful exertion. As Syme has pointed out,[15] most buildings have elevators prominently placed and attractively decorated while staircases are often bare and relegated to dark corners. Parking is provided for cars but not for bicycles, and many areas of cities have no sidewalks for pedestrians.

Fleming et al.[16] have described how the layout of units in a housing complex or rooms in a dormitory can encourage the development of friendships and hence support groups or can result in withdrawal and dissatisfaction.

Work

In the work environment, architectural layout, danger, and excessive noise (unwanted sound) all impact on stress and health. Other stressors, such as time pressures like those of assembly-line workers, responsibility for others' safety as with air-traffic controllers, nonsupportive superiors, and work overload, have all been associated with increased incidences of hypertension, myocardial infarctions, or other illnesses.[17]

Much of occupational stress seems to derive from feelings of lack of control. Among San Francisco bus drivers, hypertension was noted to be more prevalent among drivers compared to applicants and the local population.[18] The bus company management was especially concerned about their drivers' health because of the extremely high rates of absenteeism, accidents, turnover, and early retirement. The problem could be handled by treating the bus drivers for hypertension and teaching them in classroom settings how to deal with hypertension and the stress of bus driving. But this approach would not prevent new bus drivers from developing hypertension. It is more sensible to address the conditions in the environment that lead to the development of hypertension, especially as health problems have been observed in transit workers all over the world, not just in California. Two thousand drivers were therefore studied by Syme's group.

A rigid schedule imposes a tyranny, especially when it is not realistic, and the San Francisco scheduling was impossible to meet. One might assume that bus schedules are developed by individuals who ride buses and measure the time it takes to get from one place to another. This was not true in San Francisco. Instead, the bus company developed the schedule by figuring out how many buses they had, how many people to transport, and how many hours, and then allocating the buses proportionately. Thus some distances that would require 15 to 20 minutes were allotted less than three minutes and the unlucky bus driver found he was behind when he had barely got started. Furthermore, the drivers were harassed and reprimanded by supervisors for being behind schedule. Consequently, to make up some time, the drivers gave up their rest stops, and ate their meals on the go. This cycle was repeated over and over again for ten hours every day.

At the end of the day, the majority of the drivers did not go home but stayed around the barn or the local tavern for one to three hours to "wind down." When they reached home, they would fall into bed without talking to their wives, family, or friends, because they had to get up at 4 AM to start their schedule again. As a result, most marriages were in trouble.[15]

Would it not be more appropriate and cost effective to change the way in which the job is organized, and to allow the San Francisco bus drivers to develop the bus schedule? Afterall, who knows more about it than they do? They have suggested that instead of scheduling set times such as 10:21 AM, 12:05 PM, buses could run every fifteen minutes. This would be simple to accomplish, would be a service to passengers, and would make life much easier for the bus drivers. Additionally, why put rest stops at the edge of the city, where there is no one to talk to? Why not have the rest stop at the center of the city, where the driver can talk to people, including other bus drivers?

Frankenhaeuser[19] and others have demonstrated that it is not just job demand, but latitude of control in the job that strongly influences maintenance of health and well being. In laboratory tests of normal individuals given a timed task, persons reported less distress when allowed to select their own pace than when they had no control, and physiologically they demonstrated lower cortisol levels when in control. In the Framingham study, Haynes[20] noted a higher incidence of CHD among women having high job demands but poor supervision. She further confirmed these findings by an investigation of 518 women at the North Carolina telephone company. She compared operators of video display terminals (VDT) which "reflect the ultimate nonsupportive boss" with nonusers. The VDT operators had few breaks, were constantly monitored, and were reprimanded within five minutes when mistakes showed up. She reported that 21% of VDT operators with little job control reported angina, compared with 6.4% of non-VDT users, who had greater job control.

Family

Marriage is generally ameliorative for men compared to those who are single, divorced, or widowed, and mortality has been noted to rise in the year after a wife was died. Its benefit for women is less apparent, perhaps because women tend to have additional sources of social support, while many men do not. Disharmony at home, however, can be an adverse factor for either sex.

Although stressors at work imply the need for more support at home, very often the stressed individual tends to behave in a way that alienates the spouse (as with the San Francisco bus drivers) or to feel that the offered support is inadequate. It has been noted that the husbands of working wives with unsupportive bosses have a greater risk of CHD than husbands of nonworking wives or of wives with supportive bosses.[21] This may reflect disharmony at home caused by the wife's work stress.

Awareness of the patient's environment—cultural background, socioeconomic condition, work status, family situation—can provide the insight for effective counseling, intervention, and prevention. By identifying detrimental factors in the environment, the physician can help the patient to find where change is possible or to cope with the unchangeable aspects. This may prevent continuing entrapment and "hitting the wall."

References

1. Harburg E, Schull WJ, Erfurt JC, et al. A family set method for estimating heredity and stress. I. A pilot survey of blood pressure among Negroes in high and low stress areas, Detroit, 1966–1967. J Chronic Dis 23:69–81, 1970.
2. Gampel B, Slome C, Scotch N, et al. Urbanization and hypertension among Zulu adults. J Chronic Dis 15:67–70, 1962.
3. Syme SL, Marmot MG, Kagan A, et al. Epidemiologic studies of coronary heart disease and stroke in Japanese men living in Japan, Hawaii and California: Introduction. Am J Epidemiol 102:477–480, 1975.
4. Marmot MG, Syme SL, Kagan A, et al. Epidemiologic studies of coronary heart disease and stroke in Japanese men living in Japan, Hawaii and California: prevalence of coronary and hypertensive heart disease and associated risk factors. Am J Epidemiol 102:514–525, 1975.
5. Worth RM, Kato H, Rhoads GG, et al. Epidemiologic studies of coronary heart disease and stroke in Japanese men living in Japan, Hawaii, and California: prevalence of coronary and hypertensive heart disease and associated risk factors. Am J Epidemiol 102:481–490, 1975.
6. Marmot MG, Syme SL. Acculturation and coronary heart disease in Japanese Americans. Am J Epidemiol 104:225–247, 1976.
7. Berkman LF, Syme SL. Social networks, host resistance, and mortality: a nine-year follow-up study of Alameda County residents. Am J Epidemiol (109):186–204, 1979.
8. Nerem RM, Levesque MJ, Cornhill JF. Social environment as a factor in diet-induced aortic atherosclerosis in rabbits. Science 208:1475–76, 1980.
9. Seeman T. Social networks and coronary artery disease. Unpublished doctoral dissertation, Univ. Cal, Berkeley, 1984.

10. Berrveta-Clement JR, et al. Changed lives—The effects of the Perry pre-school program on youths through age 19. Monograph 8, High-Scope Educational Research Foundation, Ypsilanti, MI. 1984.
11. Wolf S. Psychosocial forces and neural mechanisms in disease: defining the question and collecting the evidence. The Johns Hopkins Med J 150:95–100, 1982.
12. Ehnholm C, Huttunen JK, et al. Effect of diet on serum lipoproteins in a population with a high risk of coronary heart disease, N Eng J Med 307:850–855, 1982.
13. Leren P, Helgeland A, Hjermann I, et al. The Oslo study: CHD risk factors, socioeconomic influences, and intervention. Am Heart J 106:1200–1206, 1983.
14. Marmot MG, Rose G, Shipley M, et al. Employment grade and coronary heart disease in British civil servants. J Epidemiol Community Health 32:244–249, 1978.
15. Syme SL. Environmental factors and the epidemiology of stress related cardiovascular disease. Presented at "Stress and the Heart" seminar, Grand Teton National Park, July 1–3, 1985.
16. Fleming R, Baum A, Singer JE. Social support and the physical environment. In: Cohen S, Syme SL (eds), Social Support and Health. Academic Press, Inc., New York, 1985, pp 327–345.
17. McLean AA. Work Stress. Addison-Wesley Publishing Co., Reading, Mass. 1979.
18. Syme SL. Socioenvironmental factors in heart disease. In: Beamish RE, Singal PK, Dhalla NS, (eds). Stress and Heart Disease, Martinus Nijhoff Publishing, Boston, 1985, pp 60–70.
19. Frankenhaeuser M. The sympathetic-adrenal and pituitary-adrenal response to challenge: comparison between the sexes. In: Dembroski TM, Schmidt TH, Blumchen G (eds). Biobehavioral Bases of Coronary Heart Disease, Karger, Basel, 1983, pp 91–105.
20. Haynes SG. Job control and CHD. Med World News, 16–17, Feb 11, 1985.
21. Haynes SG, Eaker ED, Feinleib M. Spouse behavior and coronary heart disease in men: prospective results from the Framingham heart study. I. Concordance of risk factors and the relationship of psychosocial status to coronary incidence. Am J of Epidemiol 118:1–22, 1983.

Chapter 4

Physiology of Stress

Robert S. Eliot

Introduction

There is obviously a spectrum of stresses—from mild annoyances to death threats, from momentary scares to never-ending tension—with a corresponding spectrum of responses. This section will review the physiology of stress and its interactions with the cardiovascular system. The widespread effects of stress underline the value of managing stress responses in clinical practice.

For the purposes of this book, we are considering stress to be the body's response to any real or imagined events perceived as requiring some adaptive response and/or producing strain. Stress often results from a mismatch between what a person would like to have happen and what the world delivers. In the physiologic sense, stress has been broadly defined by Gilmore[1] as "an adaptive response which prepares the organism for, or adapts it to, a given situation." Selye[2] defined stress as either positive and reinforcing or negative. It presents itself as either an opportunity or a problem, and thus is influenced not only by the degree of stress present at any given time but also by the individual's perception and resilience. Earlier, Cannon[3] also had discussed the concept of stress being the stimulus and strain the response. His major contribution to the field was the concept of fight or flight—the alarm reaction in preparation for fight or flight in response to a stressful stimulus.

From: Eliot, RS: *Stress and the Heart: Mechanisms, Measurements and Management.* Mount Kisco, NY, Futura Publishing Company, Inc., © 1988.

Raab[4] and Selye[5] among others, identified the importance of the autonomic nervous system in the stress response and later work has confirmed and expanded their observations.

Categories

On the basis of extensive animal studies, researchers have categorized responses into two or three basic patterns. Henry[6] divides the animal responses into three types: aggressive-dominant, defensive-subordinate, and hopeless-submissive. In the first two groups there is active coping, characterized by stimulation of the sympathetic nervous system, with the release of catecholamines (epinephrine and norepinephrine). In successful coping, when the animal feels in control, there is a decrease in ACTH and an increase in gonadotropins. In submissive animals, the pituitary adrenal cortical system is aroused resulting in the release of ACTH and cortisol, and a reduction in testosterone.

On the basis of human studies, Frankenhaeuser[7] also suggests three clinically useful categories which roughly parallel those of Henry. She describes them as responses to (1) effort without distress, (2) effort with distress, and (3) distress without effort. In experiments with healthy subjects performing a choice-reaction task with a high degree of control, or a vigilance task with no control, subjects reported they were pleasantly challenged by the high-control task and felt some distress from the low-control task. Frankenhaeuser noted increased epinephrine in both, but decreased cortisol in the former and increased cortisol in the latter.

In his review, Glass[8] concluded that active coping in response to a threat to status but without fear markedly increased plasma norepinephrine, while epinephrine stayed the same or even decreased.

Autonomic Activity

Activation of the sympathetic nervous system in general results in the release of glucose from the liver and free fatty acids from the adipose tissue that supplies energy to working muscles. The blood supply to needed muscles increases and the supply to visceral tissues and unneeded skeletal muscles decreases. To facilitate this process, the heart beats faster and with greater force and output. The increased volume of blood comes from a decrease in urine output by the kidney which, in turn, decreases the excretion of sodium, and increases the secretion of renin.

As Theorell[9] has explained, the acute (coping) response to stress is designed to provide the necessary energy for "fight or flight" and protect against loss of blood and metabolites. The process favors catabolism (the breakdown of substances to release energy) and inhibits anabolism (the building and restoring of tissues). Short periods of catabolism are not harmful if there are long enough intervals of anabolism for the body to restore and maintain itself. However, too frequent or long-lasting episodes can deplete the ready stores of energy and cause the breakdown of protein, and thus vital tissues may be damaged or deteriorate.

Arousal of the pituitary adrenal cortical system increases the total peripheral resistance and arterial pressure, decreases the heart rate and cardiac output, and decreases the blood supply to skeletal muscle. Cortisol limits glucose transport into the tissues but can stimulate the release of free fatty acids and glycerol into the circulation from adipose tissues. Decreases in activity of thyroid and gonadal systems may occur. These reactions enhance the "playing dead" pose. Henry[6] also suggests that ACTH and certain other substances released decrease aggression and instigate the rapid learning of new patterns, which may enhance the chances of survival. Prolactin and β-endorphin may be among substances with this effect.

Mechanism of CNS Endocrine Interaction

As described by Bohus,[10] the response to an environmental stimulus involves four levels of physiological reactions.

The first level is the limbic-midbrain system in conjunction with cerebral cortical areas. Here sensory information from the environment and internal hormonal signals are integrated and then appropriate activating and/or inhibitory signals are sent out by neural transmission.

At the second level is the hypothalamus, which translates the neural messages into hormonal messages by the synthesis or release of appropriate stimulating or inhibitory factors. The hypothalamus synthesizes neurosecretory peptides that are sent to the posterior pituitary. By means of nerves through the spinal cord, it also activates the release of catecholamines from the adrenal medulla.

The pituitary gland, which constitutes the third level, responds to the hormones both from the hypothalamus and in the circulation. Substances released seem to vary with different stimuli, but vasopressin, prolactin, growth hormone, and the endorphins have all been related to stress. Vasopressin follows footshock or emotional stimuli related to avoidance; prolactin is released from handling and novelty; and growth hormone, β-endorphin, α-MSH, and ACTH are elevated as a result of chronic emotional stress.[10]

The final level of organization includes target organs in the various physiological systems—heart, blood vessels, liver, kidney, etc. Indeed, the brain itself is affected by the stress-induced hormones, thus completing and closing the circuit of brain-neuroendocrine interactions.

The systems of checks and balances by which the body attempts homeostasis provide feedback and modulation of the reactions at every level. Inputs from chemoreceptors provide information about respiratory performance and information about pressure in different parts of the cardiovascular system are provided by mechanoreceptors.[11] Complex interactions may be skewed by such factors as genetic sensitivity, time of day, temperature, prior experience, diet, disease state, etc.

Mechanism of Cardiovascular Control

The autonomic nervous system which includes both the sympathetic and the parasympathetic systems plays a major role in regulating the cardiovascular system. Nerves of both systems supply the heart. In preganglionic nerves of both nervous systems, the neurotransmitter is acetylcholine. In postganglionic sympathetic fibers, the neurotransmitter is norepinephrine. The sympathetic nervous system acts through the effects of epinephrine, secreted by the adrenal medulla, and of norepinephrine, mainly released at the sympathetic nerve endings. Receptors for epinephrine are found on smooth muscle throughout the body and are of two general types—alpha and beta—which are further subdivided. It is believed that stimulation of α_2 receptors, found primarily on prejunctional sympathetic nerve terminals, inhibits the release of norepinephrine from the nerve terminals. The vasodepressive α_1 receptors are the predominant type on innervated postjunctional sites of cardiovascular tissues. The heart contains predominantly β_1 receptors and these are located on the sarcolemma of myocardial cells, where they are accessible to norepinephrine from nerve terminals and to circulating epinephrine. Vasculature and splanchnic organs contain β_2 receptors, and their main effect is muscular relaxation. The beta receptors are also found on leukocytes.[12] Norepinephrine stimulates mainly the alpha and

β_1 receptors, and epinephrine acts on all four classes of receptors. Except for the α_1 type, epinephrine is preferentially accepted by the receptors.

The beta-adrenergic receptors activate adenylate cyclase, thus increasing intracellular cyclic AMP. α_1 receptors produce their effects by increasing $Ca++$ in the cell. α_2 receptors inhibit adenylate cyclase, decreasing intracellular cyclic AMP.

The number of receptors of each type appears to vary inversely with the magnitude of their stimulation. The density increases when sympathetic nervous activity is low, and decreases when this activity is high. Each tends to increase in number in the presence of its antagonist and decrease after exposure to its agonist.[12] This inverse relationship may account for some differences in reactivity in different populations. For example, treatment with β-blockers results in an increase in the number of β-receptors; thus if treatment is stopped suddenly the patient would be more sensitive to sympathetic stimulation and at greater risk of a heart attack.

Density of receptors is also related to the thyroid state. Hyperthyroid states decrease the number and affinity of alpha receptors and increase the number of beta receptors. The hypothyroid state leads to a decrease in the number of beta receptors.[12]

The skeletal arterioles have special sympathetic cholinergic vasodilator fibers. These may be responsible for the increased circulation in skeletal muscles observed just prior to exercise and also for the redistribution of blood favoring skeletal muscles seen in acute stress. This activity lasts only about ten seconds, but the capillary sphincters remain open in metabolically active areas. As heat is evolved from muscular activity, the skin vessels dilate to dissipate the heat.[13]

In the skin, the veins respond to sympathetic control mainly from the hypothalamic thermoregulatory centers. Local temperature sensors can also control the vascular muscles; cooling releases norepinephrine to contract the veins and warming allows them to dilate.[13]

Overall, sympathetic activity tends to enhance smooth muscle contractility, thus increasing the total systemic resistance (TSR) and also increasing heart rate and force. This sympathetic activity is responsible for maintaining or increasing muscular tone in the large blood vessels and the precapillary arterioles.

The parasympathetic system achieves its effects by means of acetylcholine from stimulation of the vagus nerve. Its receptors, called muscarinic receptors, are found in the heart and in prejunctional areas of sympathetic nerve endings where their stimulation can prevent the release of norepinephrine from the sympathetic nerve ending. The ace-tylcholine from parasympathetic activity can also interfere with sympa-thetic functions by antagonizing the effects of cyclic AMP within the cell.[12]

The muscarinic receptors, like the sympathetic receptors, are local-ized on the sarcolemma in myocardium, are regulated by guanine nu-cleotides, and increase or decrease in density inversely to the concen-tration of stimulant (agonist).[12]

Atrial and ventricular portions of the heart do not respond to para-sympathetic activity in the same way. In the ventricles, the predominant effect is inhibition of the beta-adrenergic agonists. In the atrial tissues, the muscarinic activation has the additional result of increasing the outward flow of potassium ions which decreases the contractility of the heart muscle and slows the heartbeat.[12]

Thyroid status affects the density of muscarinic receptors exactly opposite to its effect on beta-adrenergic receptors. That is, mus-carinic receptors increase in hypothyroidism and decrease in hyperthyroidism.[12]

Thus the sympathetic and parasympathetic nervous systems inter-act at several different levels, enabling the parasympathetic stimulation to modulate the sympathetic effects for a coordinated control of the cardiovascular system.

Of course peripheral sensors (activated by changes in metabolic factors, pressure, or fluid volume) also modulate the cardiovascular system by inhibiting or exciting the vasomotor center in the brain that sends signals to the sympathetic and vagal nerves.

The venous system helps control blood pressure when volume changes. The distensible walls of the veins expand when arterial blood increases; when volume decreases, a passive elastic recoil aids blood flow toward the heart. The muscles in the walls of the veins, particularly the splanchnic veins, can contract as the result of sympathetic stimula-tion. The veins in skeletal muscle have little sympathetic innervation, and here the flow depends mainly on the pumping action of the muscles.[13]

Thus, catecholamines released in response to stress would tend to decrease the blood supply to splanchnic organs and inactive muscles, but the activity of skeletal muscles in use would release metabolites that suppress sympathetic activity and aid dilation of the blood vessels in the active muscles and nearby skin. It is of interest that Dimsdale and Moss[14] noted that increases in catecholamines with physical exercise are predominantly norepinephrine, while emotional stress induces larger increases in epinephrine.

Pathological Mechanisms

Susceptibility to illness and diseases of all types has been correlated with increased stress and life changes. Studies reviewed by Ader[15] have shown that the immune system of the body is adversely affected by chronic stress. The T-cell lymphocytes which help to combat viruses and neoplasms have been found to decline in persons who have lost a spouse. The effect appears to be a direct CNS influence, not caused by the adrenocortical effects. T-cells have receptor sites for brain peptides and also for ACTH, endorphins and prolactin. Feelings of helplessness have been associated with decreased activity of NK cells, a type of T-cell. Stress has been found to reduce the secretion of certain immunoglobulins and to affect interferon activity. Endorphins, such as those released by the pituitary, have been implicated in stress-induced immunologic changes. In addition, prostaglandin E2 and hydrocortisone can inhibit an interleukin necessary for lymphocyte production.

Glass[8] suggests that pathology such as atherosclerosis may require excesses of both catecholamines and corticoids and could result from repeated cycles of stress, probably involving periods of hopelessness alternating with periods of active but ineffective coping. This theory could help to explain the layered morphology of atherosclerotic plaques.

It is well to remember the feedback and interacting systems of the body. Pathology resulting from stress can be manifested at any point of constitutional weakness. The initiating mechanism may be different, then, from the process that sustains or exacerbates the process. Viewed from this broad perspective, the varied results of stress are not surprising since they would depend on each individual's particular vulnerabilities as modified by the strength of the individual's protective mechanisms. While studies of the direct effects of so-called stress hormones can be revealing, the indirect effects must also be considered, especially in attempts to identify individuals at risk.

It is not surprising, then, that extensive investigations of psychological and physiological aspects of coronary heart disease point toward different patterns for hypertension, angina, and sudden cardiac death, and even for subgroups of each of these.

In summary, the results of many recent investigations point to the physiologic influence of acute and chronic stress through a variety of well-known pathways. Stress is thus not a phenomenon isolated from well understood metabolic and physiologic phenomena. It is deeply interwoven in all homeostatic processes.

Dysregulation or maladaptation associated with constitutional weakness may allow penetration to a vulnerable organ system. Once the disorder takes place, its perpetuation, enhancement, or resolution depends upon a myriad of metabolic, immunologic, and physiologic factors working singly or in concert. Armed with knowledge of the physiology of stress, the clinician can often make a more accurate and comprehensive diagnosis leading to more appropriate and successful management.

References

1. Gilmore JP. Cardiovascular response to emotional stress. J S C Med Assoc (Supplement) 72:27–32, 1976.
2. Selye H. Stress in Health and Disease. Butterworth, Inc., Boston, 1976.
3. Cannon WB. Stresses and strains of homeostasis. Am J Med Sci 189:1–14, 1935.
4. Raab W. Emotional and sensory stress factors in myocardial pathology. Am Heart J 72:538, 1966.
5. Selye H. The Physiology and Pathology of Exposure to Stress. Acta, Inc., Montreal 1950.
6. Henry JP. Coronary heart disease and arousal of the adrenal cortical axis. In: Dembroski TM, Schmidt TH, Blumchen G (eds); Biobehavioral Bases of Coronary Heart Disease; Karger, Basel 1983. pp 365–381.
7. Frankenhaeuser M. The sympathetic-adrenal and pituitary-adrenal response to challenge: comparison between the sexes. In: Dembroski TM, Schmidt TH, Blumchen G (ed). Biobehavioral Bases of Coronary Heart Disease, Karger, Basel, 1983. pp 91–105.
8. Glass DC. Behavior Patterns, Stress and Coronary Disease. Lawrence Erlbaum Associates, Hillsdale, N.J. 1977.
9. Theorell T. Physiological issues in establishing links between psychosocial factors and cardiovascular illness. In: Breakdown in Human Adaptation to 'Stress'. Martinus Nijhoff Publishers, Boston, 1984. pp 188–197.
10. Bohus B. Neuroendocrine interactions with brain and behavior: a model for psychoneuroimmunology? In: Breakdown in Human Adaptation to 'Stress'. Martinus Nijhoff Publishers, Boston, 1984. pp 638–652.
11. Schneiderman N. Behavior, autonomic function and animal models of cardiovascular pathology. In: Dembroski TM, Schmidt TH, Blumchen G (eds). Biobehavioral Bases of Coronary Heart Disease, Karger, Basel, 1981. pp 305–364.

12. Watanabe SN, Lindemann JP. Mechanisms of adrenergic and cholinergic regulation of myocardial contractibility. In: Sperelakis N (ed). Physiology and Pathophysiology of the Heart. Martinus Nijhoff Publishers, Boston, 1984. pp 377–404.
13. Astrand P-O, Rodahl K. Circulation. In: Textbook of Work Physiology. McGraw-Hill Book Company, New York, 1977, 141–205.
14. Dimsdale JE, Moss J. Plasma catecholamines in stress and exercise. JAMA 243:340–342, 1980.
15. Ader R. Psychoneuroimmunology. In: Breakdown in Human Adaptation to 'Stress'. Martinus Nijhoff Publishers, Boston, 1984. pp 653–670.

Chapter 5

Pathophysiological Mechanisms

Robert S. Eliot

Pathophysiology of Atherosclerosis

As I learned while reviewing specimens of congenital and acquired heart disease under the supervision of Dr. Jesse E. Edwards, the most extreme examples of atherosclerosis were to be found in blood vessels where the intima had been damaged somehow. In tertiary syphilitic heart disease, as is well known, the ascending aorta demonstrates extensive aneurysmal atherosclerosis, and we frequently observed the paradox of remarkably extensive atherosclerosis in severely cachectic hypocholesterolemic victims of this disease. Syphilitic aortitis is known to involve destruction of both the intima and the media. Indeed, linear calcification of the ascending aorta is the radiographic hallmark of tertiary syphilis of this type. Yet cholesterol levels were surprisingly low in these cachectic individuals owing to their severe malnutrition.

Similar lesions could be found in other conditions wherever the endothelium or intima had been traumatized—from hypertension, accidental injury or surgical manipulation. The structure of the intima is like "gossamer shingles" that are interdigitated or interwoven.[1] The integrity of the intima appears to be as fundamental in preventing the lipid invasions leading to atherosclerosis as the wall of a moat would be in preventing noxious water from flooding the castle. Any rent, what-

From: Eliot, RS: *Stress and the Heart: Mechanisms, Measurements and Management.* Mount Kisco, NY, Futura Publishing Company, Inc., © 1988.

ever the cause, would allow the contents of either the blood stream or the moat to enter "forbidden territory."

New information gained within the last three years suggests the critical nature of the intima in the pathophysiology of atherosclerosis, and may alter our perception of interventive and preventive measures now in use. For example, there is evidence that restenosis occurs very rapidly after either transluminal angioplasty, where the integrity of the intima is destroyed unintentionally, or, in some forms of laser angioplasty that "boil" the intima.[1]

The endothelial cells that make up the innermost lining of a blood vessel have many functions. The cells produce a number of compounds, two of which are particularly important in regard to atherosclerosis. The first of these is prostacyclin. This substance opposes platelet adhesiveness, acts as a vasodilator, and opposes the vasoconstrictive and aggregative action of thromboxane (a product of platelets). It thus promotes homeostasis and limits thrombosis, protecting intact blood vessels. Prostacyclin also regulates the permeability of the vessel wall. The other important product of the endothelium is tissue plasminogen activator (TPA), which is the body's natural anticoagulant or clot-dissolving mechanism.

According to current understanding, the pathophysiology of atherosclerosis has four phases.[1,2]

Phase 1. Injury to the intimal layer. In human beings injury to the intima probably comes from the by-products of cigarette smoke, surges and shear forces in hypertension, trauma from catheters or angioplasty, lipid itself, or other factors not fully understood.

Phase 2. The invasion or ingestion of lipid by macrocytes within the subendothelial surface. Monocytes infiltrate and lodge between endothelial cells and within the elastic lamina, a membranous network of elastin and collagen. The monocytes continue to scavenge lipids from the blood.

Phase 3. Proliferation and migration of smooth muscle cells. A layer of smooth muscle cells lies below the elastic lamina. Smooth muscle cells tend to proliferate in the serum of clotted blood. Platelet-derived factors seem to aid this process. Pigs with von Willebrand's disease (a disease characterized by a defect in platelet adhesiveness) are resistant to atherosclerosis. When uninvolved aortic segments from these pigs are transplanted into normal pigs, the transplanted vessels rapidly develop atherosclerosis to the same degree as those of the host pig when it is fed an atherogenic diet; in the cross-transplantation, aortic segments from the normal pig do not develop atherosclerosis in the pig with von Willebrand's disease fed the atherogenic diet.[3] Platelets are further implicated by the finding that it is quite difficult to produce atherosclerosis in rabbits with thrombocytopenia, even when the intima is traumatized.[4]

When the intima has been ruptured, smooth muscle cells migrate upward from below the internal elastic lamina and continue the production of collagen and elastin. The platelet-derived growth factor stimulates this production as well as the proliferation of the smooth muscle cells themselves. Thus the atheroma can progress from a very small lesion to one that is large and obstructive.

Phase 4. Clot formation. Thrombi which are not completely obstructive may be incorporated into the plaque; they become fibrotic, more firmly fixing the protrusion and apparently accelerating the stenosis. Rupture of the atheroma may also occur in Phase 4, leading to further clots from hemorrhage and/or from platelets adhering to the exposed subendothelium.

Therapy

In animal experiments, cholesterol could be reduced markedly by the use of such agents as mevinoline which is an HMG CoA reductase inhibitor and reduces the synthesis of cholesterol within the liver.[5] When victims of hypercholesterolemia are given mevinolin in association with drugs that bind bile acids, such as colestipol HCl, there can be as much as a 54% reduction in cholesterol level.[6,7] In addition, the development of atherosclerotic lesions is reduced in rabbits that are fed verapamil as well as a hypercholesterolemic diet;[8] this indicates that in the second stage of atherosclerosis the accumulation of lipid may be blocked with this and other calcium channel blockers. Kramsch et al.[9] have demonstrated that monkeys placed on jogging programs can also have a reduction in the degree of atherosclerosis despite an atherogenic diet.

Although actual regression of atherosclerosis is hard to demonstrate, Malinow[10] has found several well documented studies both in animals and humans. Of particular interest is the observation that dietary measures could reduce atherosclerosis even when serum cholesterol levels remained above 300 mg/dl. Because the overall safety of cholesterol-lowering drugs is still in question, and side effects are common, this is an encouraging finding.

Direct observation of coronary arteries by luminal catheter techniques[11] indicates that in unstable angina the commonest lesion is a thrombus thereby suggesting that the best form of therapy would be an agent such as TPA or streptokinase.

At the present time, the laser approach to these lesions is limited to the later stages. The Nd-YAG and argon lasers basically cook the tissue at temperatures reaching 200 degrees C.[1] Because such treatment can destroy the intima even further, it may fail to provide suitable therapeutic results. On the other hand, the new excimer laser, which uses rapid pulses of energy, operates below the 60 degree C point of irreversible tissue damage, and therefore it does not cook the tissue. The excimer laser permits greater control and precision in abrasion. It also works on calcified tissue which is not readily cut with lasers dependent on heat.[1,12]

The relatively large size of some laser catheters compared to coronary arteries, as well as their relatively clumsy nature, limit clinical use at this time. Nevertheless, the approach may have a clinical potential. We practice in an era when remarkable technological developments seem almost mundane and we can thus expect many variations and improvements on this theme. Future versions may lead to safe and effective clinical use in small "coronary size" vessels. Watchful waiting appears reasonable.

References

1. Grundfest W. Therapeutic relevance of newer concepts of atherosclerosis. 55th Annual Physician's Postgraduate Symposium on Cardiovascular Diseases, AHA San Francisco Chapter, Sept 6, 1985.
2. Ross R, Faggiotto A, Bowen-Pope D, Raines E. The role of endothelial injury and platelet and macrophage interactions in atherosclerosis. Circulation 70 (Suppl III), III-77—III-82, 1984.
3. Fuster V, Fass DN, Kaye MP, Josa M, Zinsmeister AR, Bowie EJW. Arteriosclerosis in normal and von Willebrand pigs: Long-term prospective study and aortic transplantation study. Circ Res 51:587–593, 1982.
4. Moore S, Friedman RJ, Singal DP. Inhibition of injury induced thromboatherosclerotic lesions by antiplatelet serum in rabbits. Thromb Haemostas 35:70–81, 1976.
5. Alberts AW, Chen H, Kuron G, et al. Mevinolin: a highly potent competitive inhibitor of hydroxymethylglutaryl-coenzyme A reductase and a cholesterol-lowering agent. Proc Natl Acad Sci USA 77:3957–3961, 1980.
6. Illingworth DR. Mevinolin plus colestipol in therapy for severe heterozygous familial hypercholesterolemia. Ann Intern Med 101:598–604, 1984.

7. Havel RJ, Hunninghake DB, Illingworth DR, et al. Mevinolin in the therapy of familial hypercholesterolemia. Circulation 72 (Supp III):III-198. (abstract)
8. Rouleau J-L, Parmley WW, Stevens J, et al. Verapamil suppresses atherosclerosis in cholesterol-fed rabbits. J Am Coll Cardiol 1:1453–1460, 1983.
9. Kramsch DM, Aspen AJ, Abramowitz BM, Kriemendahl T, Hood WB. Reduction of coronary atherosclerosis by moderate conditioning exercise in monkeys on an atherogenic diet. N Engl J Med 305:1483–9, 1981.
10. Grundfest WS, Litvack F, Forrester JS, Hickey A. Angioscopy provides direct visualization of human blood vessels. Cardiology Product News 6(3):1, July/Aug 1986.
11. Malinow MR. Atherosclerosis: progression, regression, and resolution. Am Heart J 108:1523–1537, 1984.
12. Forrester JS, Litvack F, Grundfest WS. Laser angioplasty and cardiovascular disease. Am J Cardiol 57:990–992, 1986.

Pathophysiology of Myocardial Ischemia

Oxygenation

Normally the intricate controls on the heart's own blood supply match its varying oxygen and nutrient demands closely. However, in the presence of abnormalities or conditions that increase oxygen demand or decrease oxygen supply, an area of the heart may not receive enough blood to satisfy its oxygen needs. This is particularly true if the need is suddenly increased by vigorous physical activity or sudden unexpected mental stress. Even when a large coronary artery has been narrowed by an atheroma, the mechanisms of autoregulation (1) cause the walls of the vessels beyond the obstruction to relax to compensate, and (2) increase native collateral circulation, thereby preventing ischemia until the demand becomes too great and/or the flow is blocked too much.

The central nervous system (CNS), through a variety of mechanisms, significantly influences both supply and demand factors. Consider the role of the CNS when superimposed on the following.

Supply Factors

Obviously any factor limiting the oxygen reaching the myocardium can increase the risk of ischemia. Anemia, pulmonary disease, carbon monoxide poisoning, or any other condition that reduces the oxygen content of the blood increases the likelihood of ischemia in a vulnerable area. The narrowing or blocking of arteries by atherosclerosis, or at the capillary level, by microemboli, cardiac edema, fibrosis, etc., also decreases the oxygen supply. Conversely, the presence of collateral vessels aids oxygenation.

Demand Factors

On the other side of the equation, three major factors determine myocardial oxygen consumption. They are heart rate, systolic wall tension, and myocardial contractility. While the amount of work done by the heart (i.e., the volume of blood moved per unit time) does affect the energy usage of the heart, it is a minor consideration compared to the energy needed to maintain readiness for contraction—muscular tension—and for contraction itself. The longer the duration of contraction the greater the energy expenditure; therefore the stronger and more rapid the heart beat the more oxygen needed. Also, the larger the heart the greater the contractile load, and the more oxygen that is required. Other factors include the contractility and distensibility of the myocardium.

Singh[1] reports that hemodynamic changes associated with ST-segment depression or elevation suggest that both silent ischemia and angina at rest result from decreases in coronary blood flow rather than from increases in oxygen demand. He found that over 80% of ischemic episodes were painless and these were not accompanied by a significant rise in heart rate.

It is well understood that whether ischemia leads to tissue destruction depends on the degree and duration of oxygen deprivation. Brief transient episodes seem to be relatively harmless; however, at an ill-defined critical level, tissue breakdown occurs. Even in the absence of discernible necrosis, there is evidence of metabolic and conductivity changes in ischemic tissue which may increase its vulnerability to later episodes of deprivation.

It is increasingly evident that myocardial ischemia may not be accompanied by anginal pain or any subjective complaint. Ambulatory monitoring of angina patients has demonstrated that silent ischemia is quite common. The same person may experience painless as well as painful ischemic attacks that seem to be of comparable severity. Even when the myocardial ischemia is so severe and prolonged that it leads to myocardial infarction, it is not necessarily accompanied by pain. Among men aged 39 to 59 in the Western Collaborative Group Study,[2] 23% of all new myocardial infarctions (MI) were silent. In the Framingham study,[3] 28% of MIs in men and 35% of MIs in women were revealed only by ECGs. In women, the silent or unrecognized infarctions were not related to age, but in men they were most common in those 75 or older. The Framingham data revealed that for men the rate of recurrent infarction was the same for silent infarctions as for painful MIs. In the same study, few women with silent MI had any recurrence, but 14% subsequently experienced angina. However, the overall death rate 10 years after the silent MI was 45%, as compared with 39% for those with typical symptoms.

While reduction in the available blood supply or oxygen (such as by atherosclerosis) sets the stage for myocardial infarction, the precipitating event is likely to be blockage by a thrombus or spasm in the vulnerable area. The atheromatous plaque itself may rupture and/or hemorrhage to form the thrombus. Alternatively enhanced platelet stickiness, as from sympathetic overstimulation, may lead to thrombi which then obstruct a vulnerable area.

Angiographic studies made during anginal attacks have proven that vasospasm can cause partial or complete coronary obstruction.[4] Although such spasm is more likely to cause damaging occlusion when associated with pathological conditions, such as partial coronary obstruction due to atherosclerosis, it can also occur as an isolated phenomenon.

Coronary spasm is recognized as the mechanism in Prinzmetal's angina, in which attacks occur at rest. In this Variant Angina, ST-segment elevation is considered diagnostic although ST-segment depression also occurs frequently. Patients with variant angina may be free of atherosclerotic disease, but for those with significant coronary atherosclerosis, the spasm is often found in a narrowed segment. Both painful and painless episodes occur most often in the early morning hours,[5] and some patients seem to have a cyclical pattern. Treadmill testing is not useful in diagnosing Prinzmetal's angina (sensitivity 27 to 51%.[6]). Most patients with variant angina have normal exercise capacity but at times exercise testing can provoke attacks, particularly when the disease is in the active phase or there is some coronary artery disease.[7] In patients with typical angina pectoris, vasospasm can often be induced by emotional stress.[8]

Interacting Factors

Conduction abnormalities and the resulting arrhythmias have been implicated as major factors in myocardial infarction and sudden death.

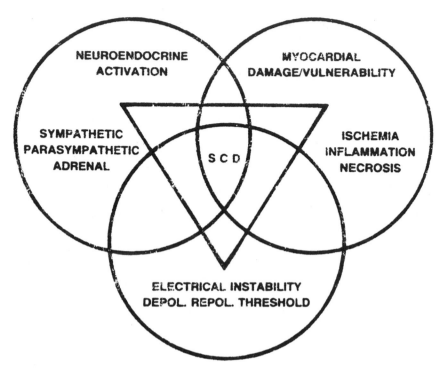

Figure 1: Pathophysiologic pathways in sudden cardiac death (SCD). DEPOL = depolarization; REPOL. = repolarization.

These in turn have frequently been traced to neuroendocrine arousal and emotional stress.

Sudden Death

Three spheres of activity apparently interact to cause sudden cardiac death. *Myocardial damage* may be effected through ischemia, inflammation or necrosis, and this "softening up" process has usually occurred on a long-term basis before the final event (Fig. 1). The second sphere of activity is that of *electrical instability* and lowered threshold to arrhythmias. The third sphere of activity is that of *neuroendocrine activation*. Neuroendocrine arousal is capable of creating myocardial damage as well as independently inducing malignant rhythm disturbances. Studies by Reich et al[9] indicate that approximately 20% of resuscitated victims of sudden death have no structural heart disease. In these cases, lethal arrhythmias may be mainly precipitated by psychological stress.

Lethal arrhythmias can be provoked experimentally in animals by electrical stimulation of the brain and occur spontaneously in patients with subarachnoid or intracerebral hemorrhage.[10] Increased sympathetic arousal also has been shown to lower the threshold for ventricular fibrillation.[11] Conversely, beta-receptor blockade or parasympathetic enhancement, or both, appear to protect against such arrhythmogenesis.

Morphologically, two forms of myocardial necrosis have been identified. In myocardial infarction both forms may be present, but the damage is primarily in the form of irreversible muscle relaxation (coagulation necrosis). Areas adjacent to the central infarct may show damage from irreversible hypercontraction, which is seen as contraction bands, and is called coagulative myocytolysis or contraction-band necrosis.

In cases of sudden unexpected coronary death, the principal lesion is of the second type, coagulative myocytolysis. This finding suggests that the mechanisms of sudden death and myocardial infarction are somewhat different. In a series of 208 witnessed sudden cardiac deaths, Baroldi et al.[12] reported coagulation necrosis in only 17% while coagulative myocytolysis (contraction band necrosis) was present in 86%, and was the unique lesion detected in 72%. Nearly half of these cases had enlarged hearts and four fifths showed myocardial fibrosis, suggesting previous injury initiated by similar nonfatal episodes.

Contraction-band lesions are also seen in those dying of head injuries and pheochromocytoma, although they are rare in sudden decapitation, implying that CNS activity is essential. We have observed contraction-band lesions in dogs given boluses of catecholamines.[13] In these animal studies, the coagulative myocytolysis appeared in a matter of minutes and disappeared within about 24 hours, leaving a pattern of empty sarcolemmal tubules. Subsequently patches of fibrosis replaced the necrotic tissue. Thus the fibrosis seen in the cases of sudden coronary death may have been the result of repeated excesses of sympathetic activity. It is perhaps of clinical interest that pretreating animals with beta blockers, such as metopralol, or with calcium channel blockers, such as diltiazem, reduced the number and extent of the contraction-band lesions.

Silent Myocardial Ischemia

Silent myocardial ischemia is usually associated with individuals who have overt angina, and yet surprisingly only one in every four ischemic episodes is heralded by subjective complaints of angina.[14] No reason has been found for the lack of pain. Obviously the absence of warning signals poses a risk; that is, an individual may continue the stressful activity without the feedback important to survival, unaware of the imbalance in myocardial oxygen supply and demand.

At this writing the diagnostic criteria remain somewhat unsettled in clinical medicine. However, there is a general belief that individuals who show significant ST segment depression or elevation (2 mm or more) during Holter monitoring, physical stress testing, or mental stress testing are likely to display silent myocardial ischemia in real-time studies. Identifying individuals of this type will, in my view, be of increasing importance in clinical medicine especially with the increased awareness that any individual with clinical angina may have undetected silent ischemic episodes. In addition, office tests may reveal silent ischemia in asymptomatic individuals.

The standardized mental stress testing techniques that we have developed over the past decade allow not only the study of hemodynamics, but the electrophysiologic features (ECG) also help to predict and demonstrate silent ischemia. Challenging patients with standard mental tests is predictive of "real world" silent ischemic episodes, as we and others have demonstrated. For example, subtracting serial 7s from 100 with a one minute time limit has been associated with silent myocardial ischemic change (S-T depression 2 mm or greater).[15] I suggest that all patients who have angina at least receive this type of mental stress test which can be performed during ECG monitoring in a physician's office. This simple test is more efficient and cost-effective than 24-hour Holter monitoring to screen angina patients for potential silent ischemia. In addition, the clinician will find that checking the blood pressure before, during, and after the stress test may provide information about inappropriate physiological arousal as well.

Physical stress testing is also valuable and of course must be performed cautiously. Holter monitoring is sometimes indicated to elucidate the precise environmental and behavioral circumstances precipitating the ischemic episodes. By knowing the precipitating events (e.g., marital discord, problems with children, friction with work associates), the physician is armed with important therapeutic knowledge.

Treatment of this condition depends upon knowing the precise underlying pathophysiologic mechanism. If there is no indication for surgery, transdermal nitroglycerine therapy has been found to provide satisfactory control of these episodes. Shell[14] has reported that episodes of angina can be reduced from 6 or so per day to less than 1 per day by the use of nitroglycerine patches in strength titrated to the individual's need. Tolerance, which has been found to occur with chronic nitroglycerin therapy, may be prevented by allowing a washout period at night or whenever ischemic periods are at a minimum for the individual.[16] Another form of therapy, less well evaluated at this time, is the use of calcium channel blockers either alone or in combination with nitrates and/or beta blockers.[17] These may be of particular value not only in the ischemia of coronary heart disease but in that associated with coronary artery spasm. Some of these agents also lower total systemic resistance and reduce blood pressure; this gives an additional benefit when "hot reacting" or hypertension is associated with systemic vasoconstriction.

Therapy for the asymptomatic patient should depend on the extent of the underlying disease. Although such patients seem to be less at risk than those with obvious symptoms, the condition is not benign. Cohn[18] reported that, for those with 3-vessel involvement, the mortality rate was about 5% per year compared to 8% yearly for the symptomatic group. He found that treatment with beta blockers led to improvement, as evidenced by objective changes in the exercise ECG.

Certainly stress management and reduction of risk factors are of prime concern in patients with both angina and silent ischemia.

In summary, recognition of the prevalence and impact of silent myocardial ischemia is changing our entire perspective of the field. Probably angina is an outmoded term. Our thinking, diagnostic techniques, and management need to be oriented toward myocardial ischemia—silent, symptomatic, or both.

References

1. Singh BN, Nademanee K, Figueras J. Hemodynamic and electrocardiographic correlates of symptomatic and silent myocardial ischemia: pathophysiologic and therapeutic implications. Am J Cardiol 58:3B–10B, 1986.
2. Rosenman RH, Friedman DS, Jenkins CD, et al. Clinically unrecognized myocardial infarction in the Western Collaborative Group Study. Am J Cardiol 19:776–782, 1967.
3. Kannel WB, Abbott RD. Incidence and prognosis of unrecognized myocardial infarction: an update on the Framingham study. N Engl J Med 311:1144–1147, 1984.
4. Maseri A, Severi S, de Nes M, et al. "Variant" angina: one aspect of a continuous spectrum of vasospastic myocardial ischemia. Am J Cardiol 42:1019–1033, 1978.

5. Sato I, Tomobuchi Y, Funahashi T, et al. Poor responsiveness of heart rate to treadmill exercise in vasospastic angina. Clin Cardiology 8:206–212, 1985.
6. Araki H, Koiwaya Y, Nakagaki O, et al. Diurnal distribution of ST-segment elevation and related arrhythmias in patients with variant angina: a study by ambulatory ECG monitoring. Circulation 67:995–1000, 1983.
7. Hopkins DG, Harrison DC. Coronary artery spasm. In: Hurst JW et al (eds). The Heart, 6th ed. McGraw-Hill Book Company, New York, 1986, pp 1009–1016.
8. Schiffer F, Hartley LH, Schulman CL, et al. Evidence for emotionally-induced coronary arterial spasm in patients with angina pectoris. Br Heart J 44:62–66, 1980.
9. Reich P, DeSilva RA, Lown B, et al. Acute psychological disturbance preceding life-threatening ventricular arrhythmias. JAMA 246:233–235, 1981.
10. Skinner JE. Psychosocial stress and sudden cardiac death: brain mechanisms. In: Beamish RE, Singal PK, Dhalla NS (eds). Stress and Heart Disease. Martinus Nijhoff, Boston, 1985, pp 44–59.
11. Skinner JE, Lie Jt, Entman ML. Modification of ventricular fibrillation latency following coronary artery occlusion in the conscious pig: the effects of psychological stress and beta-adrenergic blockade. Circulation 51:656–667, 1975.
12. Baroldi G, Falzi G, Mariani F. Sudden coronary death: a postmortem study in 208 selected cases compared to 97 "control" subjects. Am Heart J 98:20–31, 1979.
13. Eliot RS, Todd GL, Clayton FC, et al. Experimental catecholamine-induced acute myocardial necrosis. Adv Cardiol 25:107–118, 1978.
14. Shell WE. Mechanisms and therapy of silent myocardial ischemia and the effect of transdermal nitroglycerin. Am J Cardiol 56:23I–27I, 1985.
15. Deanfield JE, Shea MJ, Selwyn AP. Clinical evaluation of transient myocardial ischemia during daily life. Am J Med 79 (suppl 3A):18–24, 1985.
16. Flaherty JT. Hemodynamic attenuation and the nitrate-free interval: alternative dosing strategies for transdermal nitroglycerin. Am J Cardiol 56:32I–37I, 1985.
17. Nesto RW, Phillips RT. Silent myocardial ischemia: clinical characteristics, underlying mechanisms, and implications for treatment. Am J Med 81(suppl 4A):12–19, 1986.
18. Cohn PF. Silent myocardial ischemia as a manifestation of asymptomatic coronary artery disease: What is appropriate therapy? Am J Cardiol 56:28D–34D, Aug. 1985.

Anxiety Neurosis and Mitral Valve Prolapse

Perhaps the most dramatic associations of stress with the heart are those seen in soldiers during war, although rather surprisingly, these are rarely associated with typical coronary heart disease. Wooley[1] has traced the history of this nervous condition through its various aliases from DaCosta's description of the "irritable heart" among soldiers in the Civil War, to neurocirculatory asthenia, soldier's heart, anxiety neurosis, systolic click and late systolic murmur syndrome, to the mitral valve prolapse (MVP) syndrome, and autonomic dysfunction states. Whether these are really all one and the same is not clear; there are undoubtedly many overlaps in the diagnoses. Nevertheless, all are characterized by periods of cardiac type symptoms, usually without evidence of recognizable disease. In some cases the symptoms were related to emotional stress or exercise effort, and many patients also suffered from anxiety.

Patients with anxiety neurosis have complaints of a moderate to severe degree of dyspnea, palpitations, chest pain, nervousness, anxiousness, or fatigue. Among the most commonly reported aggravating factors are emotion-provoking situations, illness, hard physical labor, pregnancy, and military service. Dyspnea is one of the most common and characteristic symptoms, and Christie[2] has termed these cases with marked respiratory complaints "respiratory neurosis." Generally the patient feels respiratory distress both at rest and with exertion, but the degree of effort necessary to produce dyspnea varies extraordinarily according to emotional state. Sighing respirations are quite characteristic and are a helpful diagnostic sign. Precordial nonanginal pain is suffered by most patients and may be characterized either as fleeting sticks and stabs and/or dull and aching left thoracic pain of prolonged duration. The patient may relate the pain to exertion, but it usually occurs after exertion and is associated with fatigue rather than effort. Tachycardia and epigastric complaints in the solar plexus are commonly reported.

Among symptomatic patients evaluated for mitral valve prolapse syndrome, both symptoms and outcome were similar in those with and without echocardiographic evidence.[3] Possibly there are two separate conditions sharing a similar pathway of expression.

Mitral valve prolapse is found in about 5% of the general population and the majority are asymptomatic. Derangements of the valves, papillary muscle, and chordae tendinae can result in mitral prolapse. Although the prognosis is usually good, some variations may progress to severe chronic mitral regurgitation. Other rare complications are sudden death, endocarditis, and rupture of chordae.[4] Devereux et al.[5] report a disproportionate occurrence of complications in men, especially those with a previously identified heart murmur of mitral regurgitation.

While there is a high incidence of anxiety and panic disorders among patients with MVP, not all patients with panic disorder have the condition. The common denominator may be an abnormality in adrenergic control mechanisms.[4]

The fact that some of the patient's symptoms can be aggravated or reproduced by administration of isoproterenol and blocked by propranolol has led to speculation that increased beta-adrenergic receptor responsiveness or catecholamine production may be an important mechanism in the syndrome. Recent evidence favors the increase in noradrenaline production.[6]

Familial incidence of mitral valve prolapse indicates genetic factors in the primary form of the condition. Devereux et al.[7] investigated this possibility and concluded that it involves a dominant trait that is expressed mainly in females and is age dependent. They estimate the prevalence at 4% to 7% of the general population.

Greater incidence is seen in individuals with certain skeletal abnormalities, particularly males with straight-back syndrome. The differentiation of the embryonic tissue of the mitral valve and of the vertebrae occur at the same time and so the association may reflect a developmental problem at that stage.[8]

While various arrhythmias have been associated with mitral valve prolapse, they are of doubtful significance. In a study by Kolibash et al.[9] of 62 symptomatic patients over 60 years of age with MVP, 16 patients complained of palpitations suggestive of arrhythmias (two of whom had required cardiopulmonary resuscitation), 20 had disabling chest pain, and 26 had mitral regurgitation with symptoms of congestive heart failure. Only 7 of the patients with chest pain and 4 of those with mitral regurgitation had significant coronary artery disease. While most of the patients with chest pain and arrhythmias were female (27 of 36), mitral regurgitation was noted predominantly in males (16 of 26). Twelve of the patients with mitral regurgitation had a history of murmurs since before the age of 30, which suggests progression.

Sudden death associated with this condition is rare and is believed caused by repolarization changes and dysrhythmias from traction on the papillary muscle. Jeresaty[10] described the typical victim as a 40-year old woman with a history of syncope showing minimal to moderate mitral regurgitation and on ECG shows ST-T changes and frequent premature ventricular systoles. Chesler et al.[11] did not find contraction band lesions in any of the 14 cases they autopsied. In one case there was a family history of sudden death and three (of six) living siblings had echocardiographic evidence of mitral valve prolapse.

In asymptomatic patients or those with mild symptoms, no treatment is indicated other than reassurance of the generally benign nature of the condition. Stress management, relaxation techniques, behavioral modification, and other measures can minimize discomfort in those whose symptoms are stress related. Beta blockers may be indicated for some with disabling chest pain. For those with sleep disorders and panic attacks, caffeine should be avoided, since caffeine has been found to precipitate arrhythmias in persons with mitral valve prolapse and to escalate anxiety to panic attacks in those subject to them.[12] In the high risk group of men with heart murmur, antibiotic prophylaxis may be warranted, especially relative to dental procedures, to prevent endocarditis.[5]

ECGs may be advisable, particularly in older patients, to rule out other conditions and to determine the seriousness of the defect. Severe mitral regurgitation may require surgery.

Thus, MVP is a multifaceted structural disorder, with a constellation of stress-linked components under the control of the central nervous system. Managing the stress-linked components can enhance the quality of life for many and the quantity of life for some.

References

1. Wooley CF. From irritable heart to mitral valve prolapse: British army medical reports, 1860 to 1870. Am J Cardiol 55:1107–1109, 1985.
2. Christie RV. Some types of respiration in the neuroses. Q J Med 4:427, 1935.
3. Retchin SM, Fletcher RH, Earp JA, et al. Mitral valve prolapse: Disease or illness. Arch Intern Med 146:1081–1084, 1986.
4. Freeman AM, Folks DG. Psychiatric disorders in cardiac patients. In: Hurst JW (ed). The Heart, 6th edition. McGraw-Hill Book Company, New York, 1986, p 1533.
5. Devereux RB, Hawkins I, Kramer-Fox R, et al. Complications of mitral valve prolapse: disproportionate occurrence in men and older patients. Am J Med 81:751–758, 1986.
6. Gaffney FA, Bastian BC, Lane LB, et al. Abnormal cardiovascular regulation in the mitral valve prolapse syndrome. Am J Cardiol 52:316–320, 1983.
7. Devereux RB, Brown WT, Kramer-Fox MS, et al. Inheritance of mitral valve prolapse: effect of age and sex on gene expression. Ann Intern Med 97:826–832, 1982.
8. Udoshi MB, Shah A, Fisher VJ, et al. Incidence of mitral valve prolapse in subjects with thoracic skeletal abnormalities—a prospective study. Am Heart J 97:303–311, 1979.
9. Kolibash AJ, Bush CA, Fontana MB, et al. Mitral valve prolapse syndrome: analysis of 62 patients aged 60 years and older. Am J Cardiol 52:534–539, 1983.

10. Jeresaty RM. Sudden death in the mitral valve prolapse-click syndrome. Am J Cardiol 37:317, 1976.
11. Chesler E, King RA, Edwards JE. The myxomatous mitral valve and sudden death. Circulation 67:632–639, 1983.
12. Boulenger J, Uhde TW, Wolff EA, et al. Increased sensitivity to caffeine in patients with panic disorders. Arch Gen Psychiatry 41:1067–1071, 1984.

Diagnosis and Evaluation

Chapter 6

Stress, Health, and Physical Evaluation: The SHAPE Program

Robert S. Eliot
David R. Long
Jeffrey L. Boone

Introduction

Patients come to our Institute as referrals from other patients, from physicians, and from corporations. Sometimes they are self-referred as a result of having heard or read about the clinic. Initially, more than half of the patients were physicians, and they remain a large segment despite the expanded patient base. Some are cardiac patients; some are hypertensive; some are the walking-worried well; some have cardiovascular complaints such as palpitations or chest pain. Most have some form of cardiovascular, immunologic, or gastrointestinal symptomatology, often related directly to the stressors of their lives. Many come for a comprehensive health assessment and learning prescription that will optimize their performance and quality of life. Most are concerned about the influence that stress may be having on their lives and health, and they are anxious and motivated to learn how to change.

The SHAPE (Stress, Health, and Physical Evaluation) Program described in this chapter is a comprehensive multidisciplinary approach to

From: Eliot, RS: *Stress and the Heart: Mechanisms, Measurements and Management.* Mount Kisco, NY, Futura Publishing Company, Inc., © 1988.

patient evaluation designed to provide a custom-tailored health portfolio that incorporates elements of preventive medicine, cardiology, and behavioral therapy. The individual components of this evaluation are discussed briefly in this section. Some are described in more detail in other chapters.

Laboratory Evaluation

Patients are asked to arrive at 8:00 AM to begin their SHAPE evaluation. Informational materials sent prior to their visit have instructed them to fast for the 12 hours before coming. Water is allowed but not caffeinated beverages.

Blood samples are obtained for assessment of the hemogram, including a complete differential, erythrocyte sedimentation rate, serum osmolality, cholesterol profiles and ratios (i.e., total cholesterol/HDL cholesterol), and serum chemistry profiles. Serum electrolytes, liver function studies, kidney function tests, serum proteins, muscle enzymes, glucose, and a variety of other serum level quantifications are also determined to assess the possible presence of occult disease in the patients. Routine urinalysis gives additional information. Thyroid function studies, coagulation profiles, rheumatologic studies or other tests are ordered when clinically indicated.

History and Physical Examination

A comprehensive history and physical examination is a vital part of any medical evaluation. The physician spends at least one hour individually with the patient to obtain a detailed health history. The interview procedure is fully described in the chapter on history taking. Additional information is obtained through a review of systems and medications. Risk factors and consumatory behaviors are reviewed in detail. The psychosocial history, personal medical history, family medical history, and a review of allergies help to complete the historical profile on the patient. Additionally, we attempt to extend the depth of our questioning beyond the mere presence or absence of disease to issues regarding quality of life. Finally, a comprehensive physical examination is performed following standard medical procedure.

Psychological Evaluation

Every professional on our staff is trained to observe and record symptoms and signs of emotional stress in our patients. All these observations are presented in the course of the staff review as part of the overall evaluation.

To determine such things as coping skills, subjective levels of stress, life satisfaction, and emotional support, we use several written tests such as the Multiple Affect Adjective Checklist, the Eysenck Personality Inventory, the Holmes and Rahe Schedule of Recent Life Changes, and the Quality of Life Index. The Multiple Affect Adjective Checklist and the Eysenck Inventory yield measures of anxiety, hostility, depression, extroversion, and neuroticism. The Schedule of Recent Life Changes surveys the number of potentially stressful events that have occurred in the patient's life over the past year and assigns them weights to reflect their severity. The Schedule yields a total overall score as well as scores for family events, work-related events, personal events, and financial events. The Quality of Life Index essentially indicates the patient's perception of "winning" or "losing" the game of life. It focuses on key life areas including attitudes and situations that can be either supportive or destructive. Correlating these observations with other factors in the patient's health or behavior is very helpful.

In addition, a specially trained medical psychologist interviews the patient for approximately an hour and a half. This session is critical, as we integrate the medical and psychological evaluations to provide a personalized health portfolio. The evaluation, which is detailed in Chapter 11, is designed for those considered to have relatively good mental health. Patients displaying bizarre neuroses or psychiatric problems are referred to psychiatrists, as they do not fit into the structure of the SHAPE program.

A practical diagnostic interview usually works best as most of our patients are free of endogenous mental illness. Many are unaware that they are overwhelmed by a variety of life stressors over which they perceive little control. The consulting medical psychologists are very successful in assessing the subtle manifestations of specific situations or attitudes leading to excess mental stress.

During this interview the psychologist looks for the specific stressors of personal, family, and professional life. Patterns of distorted thinking and coping methods are identified and prioritized. The psychologists also determine what techniques of behavioral intervention are best for the patient, and they assess the likelihood that destructive behaviors can be altered.

This practical, non-psychoanalytic approach eases the concerns of patients who may feel threatened by the implications of psychological therapy. It is very well received.

Nutritional Analysis

Before coming in, patients have been instructed to keep a food diary for three days, including one weekend day. Our nutritionist analyzes the dietary diary with the aid of computerized programs designed to highlight nutritional excesses or deficiencies. She also determines the degree of obesity of each individual on the basis of skinfold measurements obtained during the physical examination and a computerized formula that calculates the percentages of fat and lean weight. Properly done, the skinfold method of determining obesity has been shown to be as accurate for most people as the underwater method of fat estimation. It is somewhat less reliable, however, in the older age groups.

Body mass index (weight/height^2) is calculated on all patients and then correlated with age-specific mortality data to assist in optimizing weight recommendations.[1] Basal metabolic rates, which can then be estimated are useful for some patients who have unusual difficulty losing or gaining weight. The importance of basal metabolic rates is explained in Chapter 18.

The nutritionist summarizes the findings and discusses the results with the patient. She includes recommendations tailored to lifestyle for improving the diet and activity level, where indicated. These recommendations are reinforced during the Final Summary.

Static and Dynamic Electrocardiogram

Under the supervision of an internist/cardiologist, a resting electrocardiogram is obtained. Then an exercise treadmill test is performed using the method of the modified Balke protocol. This is a symptom-limited or maximum oxygen consumption test designed to assess the electrocardiographic and functional response to peak exercise.

We look for electrocardiographic changes that would suggest cardiac enlargement, abnormal conduction patterns, or rhythm disturbances as well as for evidence of ischemia. Much attention is given to the hemodynamics generated by this maximum dynamic exercise test; that is, the maximum blood pressure reached and the maximum heart rate reached. Patients able to generate a high rate-pressure product generally are less likely to have significant artery obstruction. They clearly have good left ventricular oxygenation, the major factor limiting performance.

By taking into account the rate-pressure product, the patient's age, and exercise hemodynamics, it is possible to estimate coronary flow impairment. We use a sophisticated computer program that evaluates these and other factors to generate a coronary score from 1 (least impairment) to 25 (most severe impairment). The score helps in evaluating any evidence of ischemia and in choosing further strategies in the face of possible false negative or false positive tests. The specificity of a positive test is also increased by considering such things as the patient's physical reactions to the test, medication effects, and any abnormalities noted in the resting ECG. Further information on evaluating the tests is found in Chapter 9.

Inadequate delivery of oxygen to the myocardium would generally be signaled either by pain, fatigue, or shortness of breath. Silent ischemia does sometimes occur without subjective symptoms. Usually, however, any of three basic events can be expected to result from ischemia, namely: pain, rhythm disturbances in the form of premature ventricular beats or ventricular tachycardia, or loss of pumping function.

With the modified Balke protocol we employ, the average normal person can generate 8 to 10 METS. If a patient has achieved 12 to 15 METS without pain or shortness of breath, with a low coronary score, and yet shows an ST depression on his electrocardiogram, we would not be too concerned unless there is an adverse family history. Resting and exercise radionuclide ventriculography can often be helpful in this situation to check for wall motion abnormalities. Occasionally, we will plan a thallium treadmill test at the next annual checkup to reevaluate the possibility of actual ischemia. This prevents unnecessary duplication of technical studies.

Exercise Evaluation

The exercise habits of each patient are discussed with an exercise physiologist. Regular aerobic exercise is recommended for almost all patients. The exercise specialist guides the patient in selecting the mode of exercise most suited to his/her particular needs and interests. Exercise intensity, duration, and frequency are custom-tailored in prescription form for each patient based on the results of the exercise treadmill test.

Life-Stress Simulation Testing

The most unique part of our system is the life-stress simulation testing. The patient undergoes various mental and physical challenges while monitored by electrodes for electrocardiography and impedance cardiography and by sensors for blood pressure and heart rate. A computer connection collects the thousands of bits of information and analyzes the hemodynamics. The technician uses the computer keyboard to indicate when a testing period begins and ends, and the computer automatically averages all determinations within a period and reports these averages at the end of the test. The procedure and use of the impedance technique are described in Chapter 8.

During the testing, the patient first rests quietly for a few minutes and then performs the various tasks with a two- or three-minute rest period between each task. Except for the tilt test, all instructions are presented by means of a dispassionate narrator on videotape. This is done to standardize the influence of the technician because we have found that the attitude of the test giver can affect the results. A videocamera enables the technician in an adjacent room to monitor the patient visually during all phases of testing.

For the tilt test, readings are taken with the patient standing, and then sitting in an adjustable chair that is set first at 90 degrees, then at 45 degrees, and finally fully supine.

After a baseline measurement with the patient supine, the subject is instructed to perform the Valsalva maneuver for 20 seconds in the supine position. Next, the patient sits up and is given the apparatus for the hand grip. A quick squeeze determines maximal strength, and then the patient is told to squeeze to one-third maximal intensity and maintain this for two minutes. The Valsalva maneuver is repeated in the sitting position, followed by hyperventilation for 30 seconds.

The next two tests are mental challenges to assess hemodynamics during mental stress. We use a math problem (telling the patient to subtract 7's as fast as possible serially from 777 in 3 minutes without making a mistake), and the video game Breakout by Atari (during which the patient is to try to better his/her score on each successive game).

The last test is the cold pressor test. The subject is instructed to place one hand up to the wrist in a bucket of ice water and hold it there for 60 seconds or until it becomes intolerable.

Different pathways of cardiovascular control are emphasized by the various challenges. The effects of stress on blood pressure, cardiac output, and total systemic resistance indicate the degree of function of various components of the cardiovascular control system. The stimulation of the β_1 adrenergic receptors increases cardiac output by increasing the heart rate. The stimulation of the α adrenergic system increases the total systemic resistance by vasoconstriction. β_2-adrenergic stimulation causes vasodilation of the peripheral vessels in working muscle.

The electrical pathways of the sympathetic nervous system, both afferent and efferent, are tested by means of the tilt test. Since the baroreceptors are located in the arch of the aorta and in the carotid, a change in position from erect to supine alters the stimulus on these pressure sensors. In a normal person the heart receives more blood in the horizontal posture than in the vertical because of the aid of gravity; therefore in the vertical position, cardiac output would tend to drop. To compensate, the heart rate increases and the peripheral vessels constrict (α and β_1 stimulation) resulting in a normalization of the effective cardiac output and a rise in systemic resistance to maintain blood pressure. The tilt test helps assess the condition of the left ventricle—how well it can handle the increased blood volume it receives in the horizontal position. If there is a weakly functioning ventricle, it cannot discharge all the blood it receives, and the ventricle then dilates because of the inadequate stroke volume. In such a person with a "decompensated" (inadequate) ventricle, the change to the vertical position takes the load off the ventricle to a point at which it can handle the work, and the stroke volume actually increases. Some patients with decompensated hearts must sleep propped up by pillows to prevent lung congestion. As is well understood, when the ventricle cannot accept all the blood it receives from the veins, the blood backs up in the pulmonary veins, resulting in pulmonary congestion as fluid released into the alveoli is absorbed by the air sacs. Since myocardial ischemia can decrease myocardial contractility, we suspect that cardiac patients who get sudden attacks of coughing or breathlessness during the night may be manifesting this process.

The α adrenergic pathway is brought into play by means of the hand grip test and the cold pressor test. The β_1-adrenergic pathway is stimulated by the mental challenges. Although we expect a rise in systolic blood pressure with the dynamic treadmill test (unless there is poor ventricular function), we would not expect much change in blood pressure with a simple mental challenge. However, some patients exhibit as great a rise in pressure during mental stress as they achieved during maximal dynamic exercise. We term this physiological overreacting "hot reacting."

From a large data base of normal people and hot reactors we have found a useful indicator of moderate hot reacting to be pressures rising from normal levels to above 140/90 (mean blood pressure of 107) during either the math or video game tests or even the low challenge cold pressor test. While the cold pressor test is basically a physical test, putting the hand in ice water for a minute also involves a great deal of discomfort. It is not possible to have a pure test for each system, of course. Some α stimulation occurs in the mental tests, and some β_1 stimulation is involved if there is pain in the hand grip or cold pressor test.

Since hyperventilation disrupts the efferent vasomotor sympathetic traffic, this test indicates how much the blood pressure is influenced by the central nervous system (i.e., the mind). A patient whose blood pressure drops markedly during hyperventilation is likely to benefit from biofeedback, cognitive, and other nonpharmacologic therapies for stress and hypertension.

Staff Review

After all the tests and interviews have been completed, the staff meet for a comprehensive review of the information. Often several cardiologists are present to provide input to be used in the final evaluation. The psychologist, nutritionist, and exercise physiologist each provide unique information from which the personalized plan for enhancing quality of life can be developed. Findings from the physical examination, laboratory data, treadmill testing, psychometric testing, and mental stress testing are integrated to provide the diagnoses and the custom-tailored plan.

For each patient, a particular physician has been designated to compile the information and to prepare the individualized health portfolio. This physician acts as the coordinator in a round-table discussion during which each professional presents the data on that patient. A lively discussion generally culminates in a consensus plan for treatment that meets the specific needs of the patient. As these experts discuss the findings, a variety of therapeutic possibilities unfold.

If a patient demonstrates significant coronary disease, invasive testing to determine the extent of disease and to clarify therapeutic options would be indicated. We would therefore ask whether he was the patient of a local internist or cardiologist. If not, we would refer him to a local invasively oriented cardiologist.

For Mr. J, a 53-year-old executive with a history of borderline hypertension, we look particularly at the hemodynamics revealed by laboratory testing. A resting pressure of 160/95 confirms the hypertension. Significant elevations in cardiac output and total systemic resistance (TSR) during mental stress testing indicate that the blood pressure results from a combination of increased cardiac output and peripheral vasoconstriction. "Should this patient be on medication?" Since his blood pressure and the TSR fall to normal during hyperventilation, biofeedback is suggested. "That may be enough to control his blood pressure, and it may also help control his stress-related headaches, too." Mr. J already has a regular exercise program, and his weight is close to the desirable level. However, the exercise physiologist notes that the patient likes weight training and advises, "He should cut back on the isometric exercises; he may be training his cardiovascular system to function at high levels of TSR." The final recommendation also includes a low dosage of labelalol, a combined alpha- and beta-adrenergic blocking agent, but this may be reduced or eliminated later if biofeedback and stress management training are sufficiently effective.

Another patient seems very sound physically with no obvious problems but has an adverse family history. Two brothers both had "coronaries" at age 40; his father died at age 50 of a heart attack; and his paternal grandmother died at age 55 of a stroke. We look closely to see what risk factors we can change. Obviously, we can't change his family history or the fact that he is male. However, if he smokes two packs of cigarettes per day, and his blood pressure and cholesterol are both high, he has five major risk factors. The question then is "What can we do to get him into a program to reduce these risk factors?"

Multidisciplinary input is most helpful here as physician, psychologist, nutritionist, and exercise physiologist collaborate to develop a custom-tailored health portfolio. In this case, the plan would certainly include dietary and exercise modifications, stress management, and smoking cessation. Follow-up therapy may also be recommended to facilitate change. Such therapy is coordinated by the physician, but is often performed by the psychologist, nutritionist, or exercise physiologist, depending on the particular needs of the patient. Usually a few sessions are all that is required, as the motivated individual will benefit in a short time. Patients coming to us from other cities or countries are frequently followed up with telephone consultations. Additionally, we try to provide local referrals to professionals who can carry out our recommendations.

If an individual has many risk factors but has no symptoms and does well on the physical and mental stress tests, clearly risk factor reduction and periodic follow-up are all that is necessary. If the patient has no ischemia, no pain, and a good coronary score, the horses have not yet escaped from the barn. However, aggressive personalized risk factor intervention and stress management will be coordinated by the Center as we assist the patient's primary physician.

Final Summary

The two-hour session with the designated cardiologist includes a review of all the findings, explanations of proposed therapy or life changes, and discussion of any problems the patient wishes to probe further. The conversation is recorded on an audiocasette, permitting the patient to reinforce the recommendations or to share the insights with a spouse or loved one.

There is no set pattern for performing the "final"—it is largely determined by what produces a comfortable atmosphere for communication between the physician and the patient. Often the session starts with a brief review of the history to verify the correctness of the record. This leads to a report of the physical and laboratory findings. The physician explains what the tests can determine and what the results mean to the patient now and in the future.

The results of the exercise treadmill and the mental stress tests are similarly reviewed. The hemodynamic data detailing the mechanism of blood pressure elevation are discussed. Exercise electrocardiography is reviewed and possible false positive or false negative results are explained. The physician highlights any evidence of hypertension or hot reacting and describes how this can affect the heart and blood vessels. To reinforce the dietary suggestions and the exercise prescription, the physician may explore any difficulties in implementation, and help the patient find a workable plan.

Of course, the final also includes the recommendations resulting from the psychological evaluation. The patient's stressors are discussed, and the physician outlines and assists in prioritizing possible coping strategies. Specific suggestions for reducing risk factors, easing implementation of changes, and improving the quality of life are offered. Markers for progress and motivation are the key to compliance.

If a patient has been found to be a hot reactor, recommendations specifically designed to reduce the cardiovascular hyperreactivity would be given. This would include recommendations to moderate caffeine and alcohol intake and to stop cigarette smoking. Since smoking cessation is of paramount importance, nicotine gum or psychological intervention to accomplish this goal might be discussed.

For patients who have their own regular physician, our recommendations are easily incorporated into their ongoing care. We usually suggest that the patient return in three to six months for a partial SHAPE as follow-up to determine the effectiveness of cardiac or hypertensive therapy. For patients with no specific medical problems, we request a follow-up in one or two years. These arrangements are always discussed and approved by the patient's physician, when one exists.

Our role is to provide a complete and thorough assessment of a patient, recommend any changes that can effectively improve that person's health, quality of life, or self management, and then to teach the person how to make such changes. The AIM here is to help the individual to become *aware, involved,* and *motivated.*

Change is a must. Prevention without change, in our view, is a false promise and no bargain at any price. Once change has been accomplished, follow-up will be critical to prevent "backsliding."

References

1. Andres R, Elahi D, Tobin JD, et al. Impact of age on weight goals. Ann Intern Med 103(6 pt2):1030–1033, 1985.

Chapter 7

The Health History

Robert S. Eliot

Introduction

Myriads of medical and cardiovascular textbooks describe the standard procedures for obtaining the patient's history and performing the physical examination to get the information important for diagnosing and treating cardiovascular disease. The orientation of these texts perforce is cardiology "from the neck down." But since the focus of this text is on interrelationships between the brain and the cardiovascular system, special attention will be given to cardiology "from the neck up." Therefore this chapter will highlight techniques that reveal the stressors and support systems that may influence the development or treatment of cardiovascular disorders.

To paraphrase Osler, "given the right opportunity, the patient will give you the diagnosis." What we are seeking in particular are the physical and psychosocial factors that affect vulnerability. While obtaining the information for the history, it is vital also to establish a trusting relationship with the patient. If the goal is to change behavior, to substitute healthy habits for self-destructive ones, the key is to "earn the right." Frequently our most successful therapeutic "triumphs" are those patients who indicate "you took the time to find out who I was as a total human being and *therefore* you have *earned* the right to point out what I can do for myself." An impersonal technical analysis capped with "lose ten pounds, quit smoking, and I'll see you next year" simply does not work. Those are throwaway lines as far as the patient is concerned. Providing a list of things to do without suggesting how to do them is an incomplete prescription. As already stated, preventive medicine or health promotion that fails to build in the opportunity and motivation for change is a false promise and no bargain at any price. Obtaining it need not involve "a long day's journey into night." But there must be enough time for both the physician and the patient to develop an understanding of the relationship between the standard risk factors, the life situation and the vulnerabilities that the patient presents, whether the evaluation is for intervention, rehabilitation, or health promotion.

It helps if a member of the office staff can obtain routine information and if the patient will take various written tests that index health hazards, quality of life, and mental health. We use the Multiple Affect Adjective Checklist to determine moods and feelings, the Recent Life Changes Questionnaire, and the Eysenck Personality Inventory. Our new Quality of Life Index can also be a remarkable help in assessment.

A calm, comfortable atmosphere for the conference and examination is also an essential, and interruptions should be minimized. The physician who is frequently interrupted will have difficulty concentrating, getting the patient to relax, obtaining the necessary information, and achieving the appropriate rapport. If the patient is anxious, as many are, it is more difficult for the interviewer to gain meaningful information and establish effective rapport.

Armed with the background information on the patient and allowing adequate time for observation and discussion, the interviewer can then focus on the question "why is the patient here now?" It is critical to know what the patient perceives as the reason for coming, even if it is a repeat visit by an individual under treatment. Is it perceived as routine, to add more information about a previously diagnosed condition, for reassurance about symptoms, or for aid with some psychosocial problems? What worries him the most, and why is it worrying him? As Kleinman et al[1] and others have observed, "50% of visits to doctors are for complaints without an ascertainable biological base." Nevertheless, when understanding and evaluation are conceived as complete, the patient feels reassured and is satisfied with the experience. Thus knowing the patient's agenda sets the stage for success. For example, consider the results of allaying a patient's anxiety about symptoms or concerns that suggested serious, possibly fatal illness. Misconceptions about one's health can haunt the most stoic of persons.

A frequent excuse for not taking time for cognitive aspects of "treatment" is that it is not compensated adequately by insurance and third-party carriers. On the other hand, multiple lab tests, and complex techniques may merely compound the confusion without the appropriate preliminary orientation. Even if a time-consuming history is considered a "loss leader," it may provide a competitive edge over more technically oriented physicians by leading to more accurate diagnoses, greater success in treatment, and more satisfied patients.

Information obtained is much more apt to be honest and self-revealing under the circumstances outlined above. Indeed, the increased aloofness of some physicians and their reliance on laboratory tests rather than on the careful history may explain partly the rise in malpractice suits and the fact that autopsies have shown erroneous diagnoses or missed diagnoses ranging from 6% to 40% of cases.[2] It is sad but true that medicine is oriented primarily toward recognition or treatment of disease. During my twenty-five years as a professor, I asked the medical students to define health, and they nearly always answered "the absence of disease." Unfortunately our medical training focuses on disease rather than on "illness"—the human experience of sickness. This disregard for the patient's point of view certainly plays a part in patients' nonadherence to treatment and the mounting dissatisfaction with professional health care. Additionally, our goal is to assess the possibility for optimal health and quality of life rather than just normalcy.

The Interview

One of the most difficult things for a physician to do is to turn off the transmitter and use the receiver; that is, to listen patiently and stifle the impulse to immediately take over the interview or ask questions. Have you ever noticed that the best teachers, the best lecturers, the best physicians, are the best listeners? Too often physicians interrupt and take control before the patient has had adequate opportunity to explain the problem. Surprisingly, in the studies of Beckman and Frankl,[3] only two to three minutes were required for the patient to "unload." However if interrupted, the account could take much longer or might never be completed. This leaves the patient feeling his/her story is as important and interesting to the doctor as a lecture on papal fallibility is to the Knights of Columbus. In the studies of Beckman and Frankl, physicians tended to interrupt after barely 18 seconds; good testimony to the time urgency, need to control, and goal orientation of most of us physicians.

Patients may not present the most important information first and may actually hold back details, particularly on psychosocial concerns and areas of embarassment until they feel more comfortable in the interview. Even the Socratic, analytical approach can seem like a jury trial and intimidate and inhibit the patient. The right approach is the one that fits that patient.

Another disturbing factor is notetaking. Some patients will wonder "why doesn't he listen?" Recording of the facts can wait until later phases of the history taking if there is evidence that it inhibits the flow of information. This approach also provides the opportunity to observe critically important nonverbal forms of communication: the patient's demeanor, gestures, posture etc. which can provide important clues. A handshake with the patient not only establishes a friendly atmosphere but can indicate the patient's anxiety or apathy. Is the hand hot or cold; clammy or dry? Note the patient's demeanor, general appearance, and posture. Does he/she look tired or depressed? Neat or unkempt? Is the voice tone low or high-pitched, anxious and urgent? Is the skin color normal? Watch the eyes in particular. Does the patient avoid eye contact? In right-handed people, if the eyes are tracking up and to the right it is often a sign that you are getting the straight information; low and to the left may be an indication of deep concern or perhaps an erroneous statement. In addition, actions such as head nodding, head shaking, foot tapping, changing of facial color, blurring of eyes, changing of pupil diameter, restlessness, finger tapping, making a fist, clearing the throat may signal when we have struck "pay dirt." These observations take but a moment to note and record if we are watching for them.

In addition, the interviewer should be aware of his/her own demeanor and nonverbal communication, for this can also affect the patient. Indications of impatience, disapproval, or inattention will quickly "turn off" the patient.

After the patient has completed his statement of concerns, the interviewer can then ask questions to clarify and amplify the report. These should proceed from the general to the specific and should include the patient's feelings as well as the facts, along with the chronology of events. Picking up and repeating the patient's last few phrases reinforces rapport. Although you will undoubtedly take notes during this phase, continue to watch for nonverbal reactions. For instance, a change in facial color may indicate an area that the patient considers particularly important or sensitive.

When patients have difficulty describing their symptoms, the interviewer can try to help as long as he/she avoids leading them or putting words into their mouths. A useful device is giving multiple choice answers, for instance: "is your pain aching, sharp, pressing, burning, shooting?" It is best to use language the patient can easily understand, studiously avoiding medical terminology and jargon. To be certain that you have correctly interpreted what the patient has said, a good practice is to restate the problem in your own words, especially when the account was confusing or contained unfamiliar colloquial or ethnic terms.

In discussing sensitive areas such as sexual history, it is critical not to push an unwilling patient. Instead, a better approach is to introduce the subject in a natural way so that the patient will feel free to discuss problems of this nature if he/she desires to do so. For instance, after obtaining the menstrual history from a woman, one can ask if she is having intercourse now, and if the answer is affirmative, one can also ask if there is any discomfort. Emotionally charged terms such as "impotence" can be destructive and castrating. It is better to discuss this area in terms of "problems with sexual performance." For example, "Can you rate your marriage on a 0 to 10 scale? How about your sexual life?"

It is frequently reported that physicians have more difficulty showing necessary patience and concern for individuals of lower economic status or for older women. In such cases, a nurse or physician's assistant may be better able to obtain a complete profile of the patient's health history and psychosocial concerns.

Information to be Included

1. Identifying data: age, sex, occupation, etc.
2. Chief complaint: in the patient's own words, when possible
3. Present illness
   Onset
   Symptoms: location, quality, severity, frequency, duration
   Aggravating factors
   Relieving factors
   Associated manifestations
   Impact on patient's life
4. Past medical history
   General health
   Past illnesses
   Immunizations
   Operations
   Injuries

Current medications, including home remedies and nonprescription medications
Allergies
Exercise
Use of caffeine, drugs, tobacco, alcohol
Sleep patterns
Psychiatric illnesses
Exposure to toxic substances
Previous medications

5. Family history
Health of immediate family members
Cause of death of parents, grandparents, siblings, aunts, and uncles
Occurrence within family of diabetes, CHD, cancer, hypertension, stroke, etc. and of symptoms like patient is having

6. Psychosocial history
Home situation—now and while growing up
Educational experience
Typical day at work
Important experiences—military service, marriage, job history, recreation, etc.
Religious beliefs relevant to health or treatment
View of present and outlook for future
Sources of stress
Sources of relaxation

7. Review of systems
A checklist such as the one illustrated is useful for assuring complete information

Repeat Visits

If a patient has been seen before, the extent of the history-taking will be determined by the completeness of the earlier information and the length of the interval. The main thrust will be on changes in the individual's life and health that may have occurred in the interim, and the reasons for the present visit.

History Checklist

CHIEF COMPLAINT (reason for evaluation):

Name _____ Hospital Number _____ File
Age _____   Number _____
Occupation _____

Statement: _____

PRESENT ILLNESS: (develop chief complaint)

Interval History of Established Problems:

Current Medications:

REVIEW OF SYSTEMS:

General: current weight _____, maximum _____, minimum _____, recent
change _____, appetite _____, libido _____, physical activity _____,
fever _____, sweats _____, fatigue _____.

Integument: color change _____, itching _____, rash _____,
infections _____, jaundice _____, nail/hair change _____.

HEENT*: headache _____, dizziness _____, eye changes _____,
vision _____, glasses _____, diplopia _____, eye pain/glaucoma _____,
hearing _____, ear pain _____, infection _____, tinnitus _____, nose
bleeds _____, sinusitis _____, sore throat _____, hoarseness _____,
teeth _____.

Respiratory: cough _____, sneeze _____, dyspnea _____, sputum _____,
hemoptysis _____, asthma _____, bronchitis _____, emphysema _____,
pneumonia _____, pleurisy _____, cyanosis _____.

* HEENT = head, ears, eyes, nose, throat

REVIEW OF SYSTEMS: *Continued*

Cardiovascular: MI _____, heart disease _____, hypertension _____, murmur _____, chest pain _____, orthopnea _____, PND _____, nocturia _____, palpitations _____, edema _____, phlebitis _____, vasc. insuff. _____, claudication _____.

Gastrointestinal: dysphagia _____, nausea _____, vomiting _____, diarrhea _____, constipation _____, pain _____, indigestion _____, bleeding _____, ulcer _____, GB disease _____, liver disease _____, pancreas _____, jaundice _____, melena _____, change in bowel habits _____, hemorrhoids _____, heartburn _____.

Urinary/Genital: dysuria _____, urgency _____, frequency _____, incontinence _____, dribbling _____, nocturia _____, stone _____, infection _____, bleeding _____, prostatic disease _____, urethral disease _____, VD _____, impotence _____, sexual function _____, fertility _____.

Breasts: pain _____, discharge _____, lumps _____.

Hematopoietic: anemia _____, bleeding _____, bruising _____.

Lymph: lymphadenopathy _____.

Endocrine: thyroid _____, polydipsia _____, polyuria _____, polyphagia _____, diabetes _____, Menstrual History-LMP _____, last pap _____, contraception _____, infertility _____, abnormal menses _____.

Musculoskeletal: trauma _____, arthritis _____, joint pain _____, backache _____, pain _____, deformity _____, stiffness _____, joint swelling _____, weakness _____, tenderness _____, decreased motion _____, prosthesis _____.

Neurologic: coma _____, unconsciousness _____, convulsions _____, syncope _____, stroke _____, weakness _____, sensory change _____, tremor _____, gait disturbance _____, incoordination _____, paralysis _____.

Psychiatric: depression _____, mood change _____, memory loss _____, insomnia _____, sleep disorders _____, hallucinations _____, psychiatric care _____, suicidal thoughts _____, sadness _____, work difficulties _____, anorexia _____, memory change _____, anxiety _____.

PSYCHO/SOCIAL HISTORY:

Where born _____

Father's occupation _____

Mother's occupation _____

What was it like growing up? (stable vs. nonstable) _____

High School graduated _____

College _____ Degrees _____ Major _____

    Synopsis of highlights to where he is now _____

_____

_____

Married? _____ How is it? _____

    other marriages? _____

Children? _____ How is it? _____

_____

_____

"How do you relax, play?" _____

What do you think is your biggest source of stress? _____

_____

_____

    Second biggest source? _____

Smoke _____ How much? _____

Drink alcohol _____ What _____ Drinks/day ____ Drinks/week ____

Drink caffeinated beverages _____ Drinks caffeine/day _____

Vigorous exercise _____ Time/week _____

OTHER PAST HISTORY:

Previous serious illnesses? (childhood, liver, kidney, VD) _____

Operations _____

    _____

    _____

    _____

Other hospitalizations _____

ALLERGIES: drug _____, food _____,

    hayfever, asthma, urticaria, skin tests _____

Past major drug use (steroids, tranquilizers, sedatives, digitalis,

    anticoagulants, illicit drugs, ASA) _____

_____

Serious injuries _____

FAMILY HISTORY: (Hypertension, CVA, Diabetes, MI, Cancer)

Relation		Status	Illnesses	Age (at death or current age)
Father 1 point		————	————————————	————
			————————————	
			————————————	
			————————————	
			————————————	
Mother 1 point		————	————————————	————
			————————————	
			————————————	
			————————————	
			————————————	
Siblings:	Brothers	————	————————————	————
1 point		————	————————————	————
Hypertsn pts ———		————	————————————	————
CHD pts ———		————	————————————	————
Diabetes pts ———	Sisters	————	————————————	————
Cancer pts ———		————	————————————	————
		————	————————————	————
		————	————————————	————
Grandparents:	M (GF)	————	————————————	————
.5 points	M (GM)	————	————————————	————
	P (GF)	————	————————————	————
	P (GM)	————	————————————	————
	Paternal Aunts	————	————————————	————
		————	————————————	————
		————	————————————	————
	Uncles	————	————————————	————
		————	————————————	————
	Maternal Aunts	————	————————————	————
		————	————————————	————
	Uncles	————	————————————	————
		————	————————————	————
		————	————————————	————

Physical Examination

Many excellent texts outline the cardiovascular examination. Although the details will not be repeated here, key considerations need emphasis.

An important task is to look for correctable endocrine and brain-body conditions that may mimic stress-related states. These include thyrotoxicosis, hypothyroidism, Cushing's syndrome, and pheochromocytoma. Potentially life-threatening conditions obviously merit careful investigation.

The ultra-thin young girl or woman must suggest anorexia or bulimia, and therefore one checks for loss of tooth enamel from stomach acid, evidence of bowel purging, edema, and low serum protein. The electrocardiogram and/or electrolyte determination may indicate potassium and/or magnesium deficiency. These findings, with evidence of muscle weakness in a high achieving "perfectionistic" woman with "successful parents" must alert one to the possibility. Even the widows' hump of osteoporosis in a relatively young woman may suggest calcium loss due to bulemia or anorexia.

I always wonder about trouble at work or possible alcoholism in the new hypertensive; about marital discord in the new angina patient; about money or ego problems in the new peptic ulcer patient. During the physical examination, I try to forget the term "idiopathic"; it is a medical word-trap that precludes the expanded thinking necessary to recognize the common mind-body relationships of patients seen in daily practice. Instead, I try to see how the findings relate to an underlying organic illness or the life-stress situations experienced by the patient. In order to make the connections, it is necessary to maintain an awareness of them. What did the patient say that might relate to the physical and emotional picture? Are there nicotine stains on the fingers, nails, etc.? How does the patient smell? (Alcohol? Tobacco? Drugs?) What about bruises? (Accident? Inflicted?) Such clues and other observations increase our understanding of our patients in a total sense—neck up and neck down.

Dark suborbital circles which are evidence of melanocyte-stimulating hormone (MSH) suggest increased ACTH and the chronic stress of vigilance. Pigmentation can suggest adrenal exhaustion. Tachycardia and nervousness may be due to anxiety, thyrotoxicosis or both. In a depressed patient, slow reflexes and dry, brittle hair may indicate an organic basis for the mental condition. Or is this a case of the emotionally aggravated condition of "Soldier's Heart" (anxiety neurosis)?

Trust your own feelings! If you feel depressed while with this patient, the patient probably is depressed. Ask yourself what feelings the patient has transferred to you.

Continue to monitor speech and nonverbal behavior for clues during the physical as you did during the history. Are the patient's thoughts organized or rambling, unable to focus directly to the issue? Is there a good sense of self? The physical examination brings you closer and may bring out the real problems and concerns not voiced in the history taking. Patients expect to be touched during the physical examination and this can be a form of nonverbal acceptance and rapport, although discretion in this area is obviously necessary. The eyes of the patient are good indicators of rapport. Dilated pupils show you are making points; subtle tears underline the importance to your patient of the topic; narrowed pupils indicate anger, irritation and lost rapport, and possibly that you have lost the patient's confidence. Excessive eye-blinking may be a sign of uncertainty.

As mentioned, subtle changes in facial color are powerful clues to emotional states and to shifts in them. Increased chest breathing suggests anxiety, apprehension, or fear. If the patient is sweating, consider an emotional basis or possibly an endocrine or organic basis. Hand tremor and a tremulous voice may be clues. Does the voice reflect an emotion such as anger or sadness that is unrelated to content? In this kind of evaluation, the history continues throughout the physical examination in both verbal and nonverbal terms. This integrated approach reinforces the concern for the total well-being of the patient as opposed to the "procedure-oriented" approach; namely: "Now that the history is over, we can do something important."

Quality of Life Index

One of the unique aspects of the approach we use at our Center is the concern with assisting individuals in changing self-destructive habits and improving the quality of their lives. It has been our experience that unless quality of life is favorably influenced it is unrealistic to expect the patient to substitute better habits for self-destructive ones. Since determining the individual's perceived quality of life is essential to producing favorable change, we have developed a Quality of Life Index. This consists of an evaluation of the balance between life stressors on the negative side, and life supports (coping systems, attitudes, social supports, etc.) on the positive side.

Over the past twenty years, it has become clear that individuals who experience affective or organic disorders do not do so in a vacuum. They interact with life situations which can be associated with vigilance, alarm reactions, identity challenges, control issues, self-esteem, and other factors already alluded to in this book. The Quality of Life Index is a quick way to learn the relevance of various situations and psychosocial factors to an individual's health, well-being, or infirmity.

References

1. Kleinman A, Eisenberg L, Good B. Culture, illness, and care. Ann Intern Med 88:251–258, 1978.
2. Goldman L, Sayson R, Robbins S. The value of the autopsy in three medical eras. The N Engl J Med 308:1000–1005, 1983.
3. Beckman HB, Frankl RM. The effect of physician behavior on the collection of data. Ann Intern Med 101:692–696, 1984.

Chapter 8

Use of Impedance for Hypertension

Robert S. Eliot
James C. Buell
Hugo Morales-Ballejo

We have developed a noninvasive system for comprehensive assessment of hemodynamic factors. During the testing, the patient's hemodynamic responses to standard physically and mentally stressful tasks are monitored simultaneously via an oscillometric blood pressure unit, an impedance cardiographic system, electrocardiography, and phonocardiography. The system is effective for detecting those who react inappropriately to mental stress, and it provides a method for identifying individuals at risk before target organ damage has become irreversible. It also clarifies the hemodynamic mechanisms which are responsible for hypertension in a given patient. This permits greater specificity in treatment, reduces side effects, and thereby enhances compliance.

The course of hypertension is characterized in the early stages by increased cardiac output while total systemic resistance remains low. However, the cardiovascular system does not tolerate increased output for a sustained period of time, and therefore total systemic resistance gradually increases in response to the increased output. In this phase,

The illustrations in this chapter are reprinted from Eliot, RS and Morales-Ballejo, H: "Stress and the Heart: Measuring and Evaluating Reactivity." *Illustrated Medicine* 2(3):2–15, 1987. With permission of the publisher, Wynwood Pub., Inc.
From: Eliot, RS: *Stress and the Heart: Mechanisms, Measurements and Management.* Mount Kisco, NY, Futura Publishing Company, Inc., © 1988.

both cardiac output and total systemic resistance are elevated. Later, blood pressure becomes elevated by increased total systemic resistance while cardiac output falls, a serious and potentially dangerous situation. This is of particular concern in the presence of compromised coronary arterial circulation.

In the evaluation system we use, these phases are identifiable through determinations of impedance cardiography.

Physical Theory of Impedance

The resistance to alternating current flow is known as electrical impedance. If current is constant, impedance is inversely proportional to voltage. The value depends on the inherent resistance of the conducting medium, the length of the conduit, and the mean cross-sectional area.

For impedance determinations, a low energy, high-frequency alternating current of constant amperage is introduced through a pair of mylar band electrodes that encircle the anatomical segment; another pair of electrodes, placed inside the current path, detects the voltage changes. The current frequency is so high and the energy so low that it cannot be sensed by the patient. It is totally safe.

The system has been applied to studies of body segments that are roughly cylindrical; namely, the thorax and the limbs (Fig. 1A). Blood is the most electrically conductive substance in these areas. Plasma is considered to have a low resistivity relative to fat and dry tissue and is, therefore, the major contributing factor to changing impedance. The cardiac application of the impedance system was developed by NASA for monitoring cardiovascular output by astronauts.[1] It utilizes mylar band sensing electrodes around the proximal and distal chest and injecting electrodes on the abdomen and on the neck or forehead. The injecting electrodes are placed at least five centimeters distant from the sensing electrodes.

For our setup (Fig. 1B), the technician places the first electrode on the forehead, and the other three electrodes, in the form of mylar aluminum bands, are placed around the neck, the distal thorax, and the abdomen. The thorax band is at the level of the xyphoid process, and the abdominal band is placed 5 cm below. If the xyphoid process is rather high, the thorax band may need to be placed below it, such that the distance between the sensing electrodes is at least 24 cm. ECG electrodes are placed on the thorax forming a bipolar V_5 lead configura-

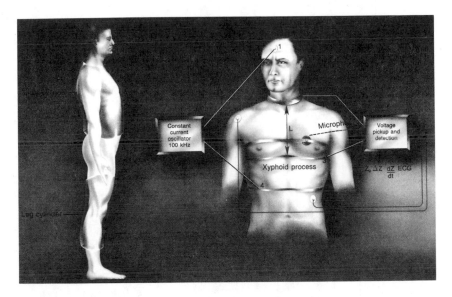

Figure 1A: Cylindrical segments of the body suitable for electrical impedance testing. **Figure 1B:** Shows placement of current electrodes (1 and 4) and sensing electrodes (2 and 3) for impedance cardiography, electrodes for accompanying ECG, and microphone for phonocardiogram.

tion. A phonocardiographic microphone is taped over the fourth intercostal space along the left sternal border for registering the aortic component of the second heart sound to determine left ventricular ejection time. The average basal electrical impedance inherent in the thorax is expressed as Z_0. As the blood flows in the segment under study, the pulsed volumetric changes in the great vessels cause corresponding phasic changes in impedance. This delta Z waveform from the impedance cardiogram is similar in morphology and timing to typical waveforms recorded by flow or pressure transducers monitoring the great vessels.[2] When the delta Z signal is differentiated to yield a dZ/dt signal, the resulting wave (Fig. 2) is similar in morphology and timing to that seen using aortic flow probes. (It should be noted that impedance cardiographic dZ/dt signals are electrically inverted for display purposes so that "peak" values seen are really minimum impedance values, but maximum flow values.) Since electrical behavior in biologic tissue is difficult to quantitate because of the many biophysical factors, the formulae used in calculating the blood flow are largely validated empirically.

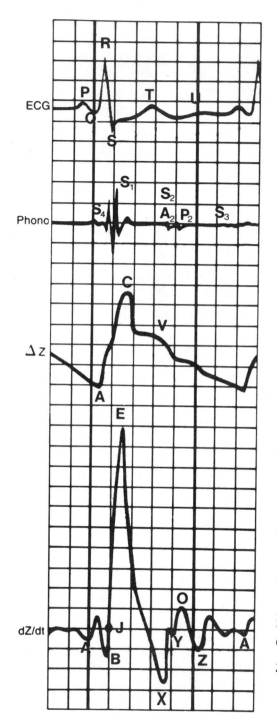

ECG

Phono

Δz

dZ/dt

Fig 2. Segment of tracing from four-channel physiogram.

ECG tracing

Phonogram:
S_1 = First heart sound
S_2 = Second heart sound
A_2 = Aortic component
P_2 = Pulmonic component
S_3 = Third heart sound
S_4 = Fourth heart sound

Δz:
A = Atrial contribution to ventricular filling
C = Left ventricular ejection that terminates at the beginning of a plateau point or "dicrotic notch"
V = Protodiastole, initiated with the onset of the second heart sound

dZ/dt:
A = Negative wave related to atrial contraction Follows the P wave of the ECG
B = Occurs at the time of peak oscillations of the first heart sound
J = Crossover point at 0 ohms/s. Signals the onset of left ventricular ejection
E = Peak derivative coinciding with the peak aortic flow rate
X = Aortic valve closure
Y = Pulmonic valve closure
O = Signal of mitral valve opening
Z = Synchronous with the third heart sound

The change in the volume of blood bears a mathematical relationship to the electrical impedance change for the segment under consideration. This constant is specific for each individual and is combined with the dynamic component in electrical impedance to reflect stroke volume.

Other individualized factors that affect the resistivity must also be taken into account. One is the hematocrit. Several different regression equations have been used to calculate the resistivity of blood as a function of packed-cell volume. This value usually falls between 135 and 180 ohms. The bioimpedance properties are also related to the relative ratios of muscle to fat as well as the inherent fluid content of the tissue in question. In general, females show higher basal impedance or Z_0 than men, and this is thought to be due to the higher relative fat content of the female body. Another consideration is the lower impedance in blood and fluids than in the air and lung volume of the chest.

Kubicek et al.[3] developed an equation relating stroke volume to dZ/dt, the specific resistivity of blood, and left ventricular ejection time (LVET) (to compensate for respiratory variation). The stroke volume (SV) is calculated as:

$$SV = \rho \times (L/Z_0)^2 \times T \times dZ/dt$$

where

ρ is the resistivity of blood in ohm-cm
L is the distance between the sensing electrodes in cm
Z_0 is the basal impedance of the thorax in ohms
T is the ejection time in seconds
dZ/dt is the first derivative of the phasic impedance change (delta Z) in the thorax during ejection time T

The following example shows how the calculation is made:

$$SV = 156 \text{ ohm-cm } (24 \text{ cm}/27 \text{ ohms})^2 \times 0.30 \text{ sec} \times 1.9 \text{ ohm/sec}$$

$$SV = 70.3 \text{ cm}^3 = 70.3 \text{ cc}$$

This equation has been used rather extensively in clinical practice. When mean blood pressure (MBP) and cardiac output (CO) are also known, it is possible to calculate total systemic resistance (TSR). A blood-pressure cuff placed on the left arm covering the brachial artery can be used to determine systolic and diastolic blood pressures and the calculations then are as follows:

$$MBP = (SBP - DBP)/3 + DBP$$

$$CO = SV \times HR \quad \text{where HR is heart beats per min}$$

$$TSR = MBP/CO \times 79.92$$

For example, if blood pressure is 120/75, HR is 72, and SV is 70.3, then:

$MBP = (120 - 75)/3 + 75 = 90$ mmHg
$CO = 70.3$ cc/beat $\times 72$ beats/min $= 5061.6$ cc/min $= 5$ l/min
$TSR = 90$ mmHg/5 l/min $= 18$ mmHg/l/min which, multiplied by conversion factor of 79.92, equals 1438.56 dynes-s-cm^{-5}

Measures of stroke volume by impedance cardiography correlate well with those obtained by various invasive and noninvasive techniques.[4,5] In the majority of clinical studies, there is good or excellent correlation between directional trends of cardiac output determined by impedance cardiography and the expected direction indicated by other maneuvers. Clinical studies suggest the correlations are less valid in the presence of valvular regurgitant lesions, perhaps because impedance reflects total aortic flow rather than effective forward flow. The magnitude of dZ/dt is undoubtedly the result of a velocity factor as well as a volume component and this may somewhat impair absolute volume calculations. When there is great variance among serial determinations by invasive techniques and/or great variance of morphology or magnitude of impedance waveforms, the determination of stroke volume by impedance cardiography is unreliable. Otherwise, in our experience, stroke volume obtained by impedance cardiography is as accurate as, and agrees with, that obtained by invasive methods. Even in the presence of valvular regurgitation, qualitative and directional information of aortic flow may be correct, although the calculated stroke volume may be skewed.[2]

In our study[6] we found the correlation of this method with thermodilution techniques to be about .73, but if valvular disease is eliminated the correlation is higher—about .80 in our study and .86 in that of Goldstein et al.[5]

Our protocol for impedance cardiography includes a computer program that converts the R-R interval to heart rate (HR) on each beat, and stroke volume (SV) is measured on a beat-to-beat basis and indexed by body surface to yield the stroke volume index. The blood pressure monitor automatically samples systolic blood pressure (SBP), diastolic blood pressure (DBP), and mean arterial blood pressure (MBP) for each task and transmits this information to the computer. For every beat, the computer uses the last available MBP and the current heart rate and stroke volume to calculate total systemic resistance (TSR) as previously described.

As backup, ECG, delta Z, dZ/dt, and heart sounds are recorded on a 4-channel physiograph (see Fig. 2). Because of the considerable shift in dZ/dt as a function of respiration, samples should always be taken during the same phase of respiration each time or, alternatively, all samples throughout respiration for a full 60 seconds should be measured and averaged.

In general, since Z_0 is inversely related to thoracic fluid accumulation, it will be higher in the erect than in the supine position and decreases as fluid accumulates in the thorax.

Stress Testing

The Life Stress Simulation testing we have developed measures the physiologic responses to mild stresses that are similar to those encountered in daily activities. The most fundamental of these tests is a modified tilt test during which ventricular function is examined. Hemodynamics, including stroke volume and total systemic resistance, are calculated during lesser (erect) and greater (supine) amounts of preload. The patient is studied while standing and then in a reclining chair that is tilted progressively from 90 degrees to 45 degrees to supine. Mental tests are a video game and serial subtraction. Additional challenges are hyperventilation, Valsalva maneuver, handgrip, and the cold pressor test.

The computer obtains thousands of bits of information per second on what is happening with the cardiovascular system. It can give us an immediate printout of cardiac output, total systemic resistance, stroke volume, vascular rigidity, and other information that identifies the type of disorder and indicates the proper management, both pharmacologic and nonpharmacologic.

Ambulatory monitoring shows that responses to real-life events are closely reflected by laboratory life-stress testing.[7]

Types of Reactivity

Since Blood Pressure = Flow × Resistance, only three possible combinations of flow and resistance can yield an increase in blood pressure. Blood pressure can be elevated exclusively by cardiac output while total systemic resistance remains unchanged or even drops slightly (output reactors). Blood pressure can be elevated exclusively through vasoconstriction with cardiac output unchanged or lower (vasoconstrictive reactors). Or blood pressure can rise from contributions of both output and resistance (combined reactors).

The testing we have devised addresses all three factors of the blood pressure equation—BP, CO, and TSR—and establishes the basic mechanisms of blood pressure elevation or reactivity. We have also devised a graphic method of showing the changes in MBP in relation to changes in the other two components (CO and TSR). With MBP as the Y axis, and CO as the X axis, we obtain regression lines for TSR (Fig. 3) by substituting values in the blood pressure equation. Thus, if MBP is 80 mmHg and CO is 8 l/min, point Z will represent a TSR of 10 mmHg/l/min or 799.2 dynes-s-cm^{-5}. The point Z' also represents a TSR of 10 mmHg/l/min, the result of dividing MBP of 120 by CO of 12. The other lines are obtained in a similar manner.

The changes generated as a result of the tests can be shown as vectors from the resting value. This graphically demonstrates whether the patient is reacting normally or is a vasoconstrictive, output, or combined reactor. In Figure 4, Vector A shows the response of a normal reactor. At rest, while sitting (S), his blood pressure was 110/70 (MBP = 83); CO was 7.4 l/min; and TSR equaled 900 dynes-s-cm. When challenged by playing a video game (G), his reactions were within normal limits with values of blood pressure at 135/85 (MBP = 102); CO at 9.3 l/min; and TSR at 869 dynes-s-cm^{-5}.

Vector B in Figure 4 shows results of an output reactor. The elevation in blood pressure in response to stress is due to an increase in cardiac output from 8 l/min to 11 l/min. Vector C is an example of a combined reactor; the increase in blood pressure from a mean of 93 to 118 is due to increases in both CO (from 7.4 to 7.9 l/min) and TSR (from 1000 to 1200 dynes-s-cm^{-5}). Example D clearly shows the vasoconstrictive response pattern with the vector oriented leftward toward the higher levels of TSR. From a resting level (S) of 97 mmHg for MBP and 1100 dynes-s-cm^{-5} for TSR, this patient responded with increases to 123 mmHg and 1966 dynes-s-cm^{-5} respectively.

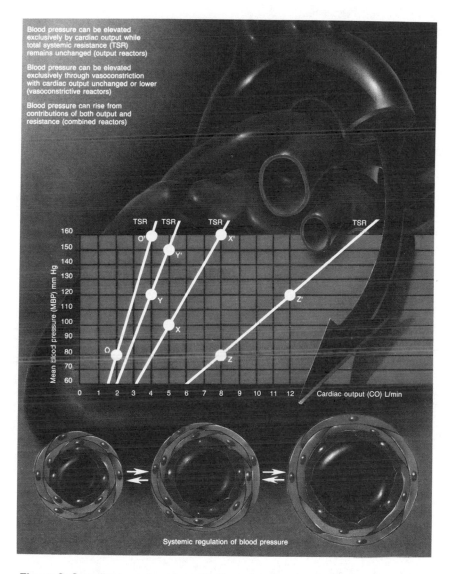

Figure 3: Coordinate system for patient graphs showing derivation of regression lines for total systemic resistance (TSR).

The parameters indicate the stage of hypertensive disease. Early in the disease, at least in Caucasians, there is an increased adrenergic drive with increased plasma renin activity, elevated stroke volume index, and

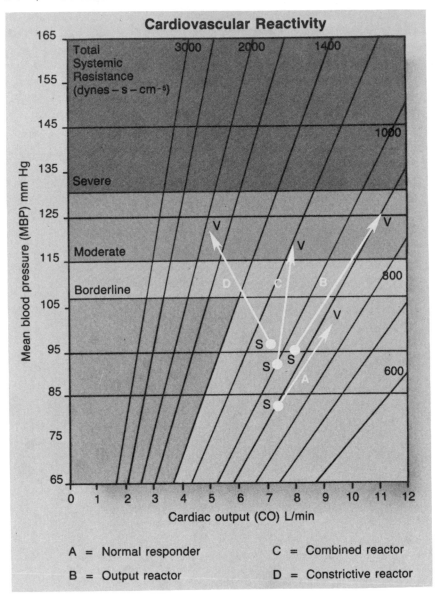

Figure 4: Vector lines indicating cardiovascular responses of four patients while sitting at rest (S) and while playing a video game (V).

elevated heart rate; total systemic resistance will tend to be normal or low; and central blood volume will tend to be expanded. Later in the course of the illness, the total systemic resistance will gradually increase with a concomitant drop in cardiac index, and a contraction of plasma volume.

In pure hypertension, hemodynamic analysis allows us to select the agent that is appropriate to the underlying cause; that is, whether the blood pressure is being raised by changes in output, changes in resistance, or both. We therefore use less medication, patients have fewer side effects, and compliance is enhanced. In the output hypertensive, nonpharmacologic management may suffice.

In our Life Stress Simulation laboratory we have found that serial subtraction and the video game tend to be beta-mediated tasks. Normally patients will vasodilate or show no change in total systemic resistance during these tasks. If blood pressure rises, it is usually due to cardiac output mechanisms.

The cold pressor test appears to be a vasoconstrictive or alpha-mediated task. Here we expect to see some increase in vasoconstriction. In some subjects, the cardiac output may drop because of depressed stroke volume index. Although the cold pressor reflex is alpha-adrenergic mediated and a spinal reflex, higher cortical functions and emotions, such as fear or pain, may activate beta-adrenergic pathways as well, resulting in a decreased or absent vasoconstrictive response. Such subjects may actually show an increase in their cardiac output, primarily through tachycardia and beta-adrenergic influences. However, the usual cold pressor response demonstrates vasoconstriction and no change in heart rate, or a slight drop due to baroreceptor activation from increased pressure.

Hyperventilation shows the degree to which blood pressure is maintained by vasomotor center sympathetic drive. Because hyperventilation depresses efferent traffic from the vasomotor center, it blocks the stress-caused stimulation of the sympathetic system. This generally results in increased cardiac output and a drop in TSR through vasodilation. Patients showing a marked drop in TSR with this test are likely to benefit from behavioral techniques such as biofeedback for blood pressure control.

Treatment

Hypertensives and hot reactors can be treated according to the mechanism by which the blood pressure is elevated. Output reactors respond to beta blockade. Combined reactors may benefit from a moderate dose of a beta blocker and a vasodilator to lower total systemic resistance. Vasoconstrictive reactors appear to be at the highest risk and therefore are of the greatest concern. Because these individuals cannot increase their cardiac output, they require immediate study by invasive techniques. Many have critical lesions that account for "pump failure." When no underlying mechanism is found, vasodilatory afterload therapy is certainly indicated.

For some, especially those with elevated output, behavioral therapy can minimize further damage. In many cases, pharmacological therapy may not even be necessary. Because cardiovascular damage generally results from the interaction of the risk factors rather than from any factor alone, risk factor reduction is beneficial. Biofeedback training, relaxation therapy, and stress management also have been found to reduce blood pressure and reactivity.

Case Studies

As previously discussed, about one in five apparently healthy individuals reveal an extreme cardiovascular arousal to simple mental tasks. Inappropriate arousal or hot reacting in the laboratory correlates well with average blood pressure determination during real-life activity at work and at home. As Devereaux et al.[8] have demonstrated, it is this blood pressure that determines the risk of future target organ damage.

Here is an example of one of our early patients, a financial planner under treatment for hypertension. He did very well on the treadmill; blood pressure rose to 175/85. However, when asked to subtract sevens serially from 777 without mistake, his pressure rose to 171/95, almost as high in the systolic and higher in the diastolic. This person appeared very cool on the surface but below the surface he acted as if he were fighting saber-toothed tigers thirty or forty times a day. This case demonstrates the importance of knowing not only the resting blood pressure but also the blood pressure obtained while the patient is mentally challenged. When this individual was monitored for 72 hours, we confirmed that his blood pressure levels at work were at least as high, and at times even higher, than what we had noted with a simple mental task in our laboratory setting.

We have followed up on a number of such "hot reactors" to determine whether this characteristic has prospective implications, as the literature on hypertension suggested. Rose[9] had noted that air traffic

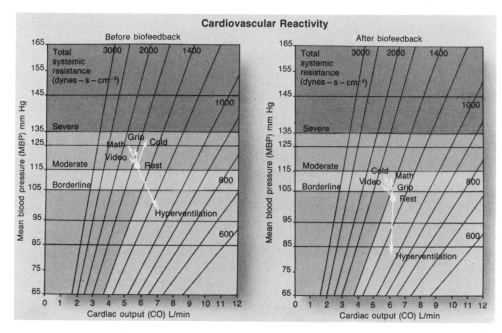

Figure 5: Cardiovascular reactivity before biofeedback training and after biofeedback training of same patient.

controllers who had normal blood pressure at rest but had elevated blood pressure while on active duty in the tower became hypertensive within three years. Falkner et al.[10] found that normotensive children of hypertensive parents were more reactive to stress than other normotensives. Theorell[11] noted that identical twins can show different reactivities and that the more reactive twin develops the infarction. We demonstrated that among individuals who have had heart attacks, independent of whether they were type A or type B, those who were hot reactors were most likely to have reinfarction within two years.[12]

Another healthy individual, who was a key executive of a major corporation, came for a complete evaluation. Because he exercised daily, he was physically fit and did very well on the treadmill, his clinical, electrocardiographic, and blood pressure responses to exercise were normal, and his functional capacity was excellent. However, during the math stress test his blood pressure rose to 176/100 (MBP = 125) with an increase in TSR to 1816.4 dynes-s-cm^{-5} (normal is about 1200 dynes-s-cm^{-5}) and a drop in cardiac output from 5.7 to 5.5 l/min. During the cold pressor test his blood pressure rose to 172/105 (MBP = 127) due mainly to cardiac output increasing to 6.3 l/min. Figure 5 shows the graph of his hemodynamic responses. Since the hyperventilation test indicated that his blood pressure was largely driven by vasomotor center sympathetic stimulation, he was given training in biofeedback for blood pressure control. Figure 5 also shows the improvements after he had completed three two-hour biofeedback training sessions. His blood pressure during the math test dropped from 176/100 before therapy to 153/90, and the TSR dropped from 1816.4 to 1503.6 dynes-s-cm^{-5}.

The next example clearly shows the effect of a beta-blocking agent on a hypertensive whose hyperreactivity resulted from increased cardiac output. When we tested him in our lab, his resting blood pressure was slightly elevated at 166/85 (MBP 112) with a cardiac output of 5.9 l/min and a TSR of 1517.1 dynes-s-cm^{-5}. During the video game his blood pressure shot up to 196/107 (MBP 137) with an increase in cardiac output to 7.4 l/min. We prescribed the beta blocker nadolol, and retested him two months after the start of therapy. At the retest (Fig. 6), his resting MBP had dropped from 112 to 91, and during the video game it was now 107, compared to 137 before treatment. His cardiac output at rest was unchanged, but during the video game playing it was now only 5.1 l/min.

Another significant case was a dentist who liked to jog. His day included an hour or more of jogging morning and evening. His baseline blood pressure was 106/64, but his TSR was elevated to 2343 dynes-s-cm^{-5}. Also his serum cortisol level was high. Because more than 30 minutes a day of jogging is not therapeutic, we felt he was jogging too much. With the aid of the data, we were able to persuade him to cut back to a half hour per day. We also taught him a variety of relaxation techniques which aided his sleep. Some serious domestic problems that he was literally running away from were also addressed. As he got his life in order, his state of vigilance disappeared and his total systemic resistance dropped. He did not require any medication.

Hemodynamic evaluation is also useful for determining the effectiveness of medication. A patient who was taking propanolol 120 mg/day, seemed to have achieved good control, with a resting blood pressure of 148/80, although his TSR was slightly elevated at 1470.0 dynes-s-cm^{-5}. However, during the stress of the mental arithmetic test, his blood pressure rose to 166/85 (MBP 112) with an increase in TSR to 1864.8 dynes-s-cm^{-5}. As an accountant, he makes his living with mathematics, and it is evident that his blood pressure would be elevated most of the day. The propanolol achieved what we call "cosmetic" control, but the real-time blood pressure would correlate with his response to the math test. We changed his medication to labetalol which has both

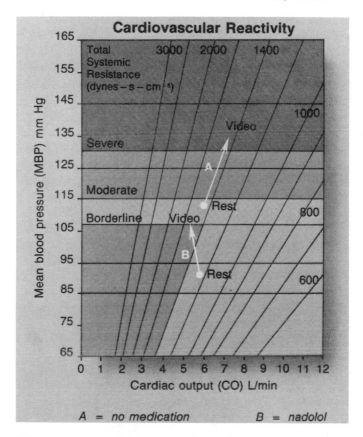

Figure 6: Hemodynamics of a hyperreactive patient before treatment and after two months on the beta blocker nadolol.

beta- and alpha-adrenergic blocking effects. On retest two months later, his blood pressure at rest was lower, being 128/75 (MBP 93) as a result of the lower TSR of 1327.2 dynes-s-cm^{-5}. His response to the math test also revealed a marked improvement as can be seen in Figure 7.

Another example is a 53-year-old man who was on various medications. His baseline blood pressure was 158/85, but his resistance was elevated. In the ultimate challenge for him—the cold pressor test—his blood pressure went up to 181/109, and the TSR increased to about five times what it ought to be. But more importantly, his stroke volume faded to such a low point that it was practically indeterminable—it was beyond the credible measurement system. We were very concerned because he fit into the third hemodynamic pattern, of raised total sys-

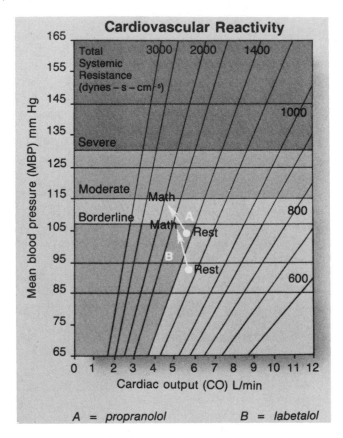

Figure 7: Responses of hypertensive patient first treated with the beta blocker propanolol and then treated for two months with labetalol which has both alpha- and beta-blocking effects.

temic resistance and diminished cardiac output. Such individuals, in our experience, are potential victims of sudden cardiac death or some other related disaster. We tried to get him back for further study to determine whether there was a critical lesion or at least to provide medication to reduce his total systemic resistance or unload the left ventricle. Unfortunately, he said he was too busy to return, especially as he didn't feel bad, and within two months of the test he was found dead at his desk. He's the only one we have lost with these vasoconstrictive hemodynamics in the past five years. We now deal with these conditions either by interventive invasive techniques or with appropriate afterload therapy (unloading the left ventricle).

Thus, utilization of the hemodynamic profile can permit hypertensive treatment to be custom-tailored to the underlying physiologic state and adjusted according to hemodynamic changes not apparent from blood pressure alone. In addition, the amount of medication can be kept at a minimum. This aids in avoiding side effects and in gaining patient adherence over rather long periods of time.

We can now obtain hemodynamic data equivalent to a heart catheterization in a comfortable, noninvasive, cost-effective manner. The data reveal the hemodynamic mechanisms allowing the precise selection of pharmacologic agents suited to the hemodynamic conditions. Unpleasant direct effects of antihypertensive therapy can result from administering a hemodynamically inappropriate agent. Thus, pharmacologic misadventures can be predicted and avoided by hemodynamic testing, and the reduced incidence of side effects enhances compliance. Prognostic indices can be developed on the basis of the hemodynamic patterns; and by utilizing mental stress tests, additional critical information regarding real-time blood pressure and potential target organ illness is obtained readily, accurately, and inexpensively. Control is hemodynamic, not just cosmetic.

References

1. Kubicek WG, Karnegis JN, Patterson RP, et al. Development and evaluation of an impedance cardiac output system. *Aerosp Med* 37:1208–1212, 1966.
2. Buell JC. Impedance cardiography and plethysmography. In: Herd JA, Gotto AM, Kaufmann PG, et al. (eds). Cardiovascular Instrumentation: Applicability of New Technology to Biobehavioral Research. NIH publication No. 84-1654, 1984, pp 227–238.
3. Kubicek WG, Kottke FJ, Ramos MU, et al. The Minnesota impedance cardiograph—theory and applications. *Biomedical Eng* 9:410–416, 1974.
4. Ebert TJ, Eckberg DL, Vetrovec GM, et al. Impedance cardiograms reliably estimate beat-by-beat changes of left ventricular stroke volume in humans. *Cardiovasc Res* 18:354–360, 1984.
5. Goldstein DS, Cannon RO III, Zimlichman R, et al. Clinical evaluation of impedance cardiography. *Clin Physiol* 6:235–251, 1986.
6. Buell JC, McKinney ME, Muers D, et al. The validity of impedance cardiology (abstr). *Psychophysiology* 20:420, 1983.
7. McKinney ME, Miner MH, Ruddel H, et al. The standardized mental stress test protocol: test-retest reliability and comparison with ambulatory blood pressure monitoring. *Psychophysiology* 22:453–463, 1985.
8. Devereux RB, Pickering TG, Harshfield GA, et al. Left ventricular hypertrophy in patients with hypertension: importance of blood pressure response to regularly recurring stress. *Circulation* 68:470–476, 1983.

9. Rose RM, Jenkins CD, Hurst MW. Air traffic controller health change study: a prospective investigation of physical, psychological and work-related changes. National Technical Information Service (FAA-AM-78-39), Springfield, VA, 1978.

10. Falkner B, Onesti G, Hamstra B. Stress response characteristics of adolescents with high genetic risk for essential hypertension: a five-year follow-up. *Clin Exp Hypertens* 3:583–591, 1981.

11. Theorell T, de Faire U, Schalling D, et al. Personality traits and psychophysiological reactions to a stressful interview in twins with varying degrees of coronary heart disease. *J Psychosom Res* 23:89–99, 1979.

12. Sime WE, Buell JC, Eliot RS. Cardiovascular responses to emotional stress (quiz interview) in post-myocardial infarction patients and matching control subjects. *J Hum Stress* 3:39–46, 1980.

Chapter 9

Treadmill Testing and the Exercise Prescription

Robert S. Eliot
Hugo Morales-Ballejo

Exercise Testing

Preliminaries

Exercise testing such as the treadmill test has four main purposes: for diagnosis, evaluation of treatment, determination of different variables for the exercise prescription, and the determination of functional capacity and/or severity of disease. Before ordering the test, the physician should know which of these purposes the test is to serve and what use will be made of the results, both unexpected findings as well as expected ones.

To assure the patient's safety, the personnel should be well trained and experienced in exercise testing and must also be trained in CPR and in related emergency procedures. Defibrillating equipment must also be available nearby.

Before the testing session, the physician performing the test needs to be familiar with the participant's relevant past and present medical history, with particular emphasis on cardiovascular events to determine whether any of the contraindications for exercise are present. This is necessary to prevent the testing of unsuitable patients as well as to

From: Eliot, RS: *Stress and the Heart: Mechanisms, Measurements and Management.* Mount Kisco, NY, Futura Publishing Company, Inc., © 1988.

permit proper interpretation of the results. It is important to note what medications the patient has taken and whether there are metabolic problems such as reduced potassium or magnesium which can cause a false positive electrocardiographic response. It is critical to know why the test is being done; that is, what is being sought diagnostically that will influence prognosis and/or management.

Prior to the testing day, patients should be advised as to suitable clothing and instructed not to smoke, eat or drink for 4 hours before the test. (Meals and glucose ingestion can cause false positives and will increase the risk in patients with myocardial ischemia.) It is also advisable to provide patients with an explanation of the test procedures including a description of the possible risks and discomforts and potential benefits to be expected. Whether medications should be stopped will depend on the purpose of the test and the type of medications being used.

Before the actual exercise testing, 12-lead ECGs are taken in supine and standing positions and post-hyperventilation. These maneuvers may produce labile ST-T changes that can help in the interpretation of the exercise ECG.

Those Who Should Not Have an Exercise Test

The following are contraindications for maximal exercise testing (Modification of ACSM Guidelines).[1]

1. Recent acute myocardial infarction. Sometimes a submaximal test is performed during the resolution of a myocardial infarction prior to the discharge of the patient from the hospital. This would be limited to patients recovering from uncomplicated infarction with no clinically significant abnormalities.[2]
2. Angina pectoris of recent onset or rapidly progressive with recent electrocardiographic changes.
3. Cardiac failure and complete atrioventricular block.
4. Acute or subacute myocarditis.
5. Severe aortic or subaortic stenosis.
6. Severe arrhythmias (ventricular tachycardia, paroxysmal supraventricular tachycardia)
7. Dissecting aneurysms.
8. Pulmonary embolism.
9. Severe anemia.
10. Recent or active infectious episodes.

11. Uncontrolled metabolic disease.
12. Neuromuscular or musculoskeletal orthopedic or arthritic disorders that could prevent activity.
13. Other conditions such as complications of pregnancy, psychoneurotic disturbances, excessive medication effects.

Physiology of Exercise Testing

The aim of the exercise test is to progressively overload the cardiovascular system in order to reveal abnormalities not present at rest. It also permits the evaluation of functional aerobic power or maximum oxygen uptake (VO_2 max).

VO_2 is generally estimated from standardized tests administered on a treadmill, cycle ergometer, or steps. Several protocols can be used for diagnostic purposes and for the determination of VO_2 max. All of them start with low levels of effort and continue with progressively higher levels. When exercise begins, the oxygen intake does not immediately meet demands and energy is acquired anaerobically. Oxygen intake matches demand after 2 to 4 minutes of exercise, and exercise can continue as long as the energy requirements are met. If aerobic processes to provide energy are exhausted, anaerobic processes are used, leading to the production of lactic acid which must be oxidized after exercise is terminated. After exercise, the oxygen intake returns slowly to resting levels. Recovery of oxygen intake in excess of resting needs is called the "oxygen debt."[3]

The VO_2, indicating the metabolic costs of activities, is often measured in METs; a MET represents the approximate rate of oxygen expenditure used while sitting quietly, and is equal to 3.5 ml O_2/min/kg of body weight. VO_2 in METs for exercise is determined by dividing the metabolic rate during exercise by the metabolic rate at rest. (For example: if the metabolic cost for a level of exercise is 21 ml O_2/kg/min, then 21 divided by 3.5 [the VO_2 at rest] equals 6 METs.) The MET cost of treadmill exercise is independent of body weight. The MET cost of bicycle ergometry is dependent on body weight because the oxygen cost of cycling is related to the resistance of pedaling regardless of body weight.[1] The net cost will be higher in individuals with lower weight because their VO_2 at rest is less. METs may be estimated from the intensity of the exercise performed or by calculating oxygen uptake from measurements of per minute ventilation and expired gas composition. Either method may be used to evaluate the exercise test and to determine the exercise prescription.

Maximum VO_2 (VO_2 max) is equal to maximum cardiac output (CO) times maximum arteriovenous oxygen difference (AVO_2), which is the amount of O_2 being taken from the arterial blood by the body tissues. VO_2 Max $= CO \times AVO_2$.

Cardiac output is equal to the product of stroke volume (SV) and heart rate (HR). $CO = SV \times HR$.

Stroke volume rises during exercise, reaching a plateau at a relatively low work load, and further increases in cardiac output are then due to changes in heart rate alone. Therefore the exercise heart rate is a good indicator of both cardiac output and the energy expenditure during exercise. Furthermore, heart rate is a major determinant of myocardial oxygen consumption (MVO_2), together with intramyocardial wall tension (left ventricular pressure $\times$ end diastolic volume) and contractility.

Since systolic blood pressure (SBP) is an expression of left ventricular pressure, the product of heart rate and systolic blood pressure (double product) provides an estimate of myocardial oxygen consumption (tension-time indices) and is a very good noninvasive method for determining this value. However, in patients with a previous myocardial infarction, this index is not always applicable as an expression of MVO_2, because increased myocardial wall tension may result in an increase in myocardial consumption disproportionate to the heart rate.[4] Morales has found that patients with ventricular dysfunction may have a hypertensive response to exercise.

Testing Protocol

Treadmill testing is the most common method of testing and the Bruce protocol is the most widely used. Basically, it starts at 1.7 mi/hr at a 10% grade and is increased in speed and incline every three minutes. Other protocols used are Balke, Naughton, and Ellestad. Since these protocols have different rates of increase in workloads (VO_2 or METS) they cannot be compared with regard to duration of testing. However, the maximum workloads will be similar regardless of the protocol. For example, in the Bruce protocol, which has a more abrupt increase in workload, during the sixth minute of exercise the VO_2 will be approximately 7 METS, but in the sixth minute of the Naughton protocol, the

VO_2 will be only 3 METS. The Bruce protocol increases approximately 3 METS in each 3-minute stage, while the Naughton protocol increases 1 MET each 2-minute stage.

Selection of the protocol depends on the characteristics of the patient, the purpose of the test, and the preference of the person conducting the test. In general, any continuous multistage test that starts at a low MET level (2 to 3 METS), has 1- to 3-minute stages, and increases the workload by no more than 1 to 3 METs per stage can be adapted for almost all individuals. In our laboratory, we use a modified Balke protocol. This test allows 2 minutes for a warm-up and general cardiovascular respiratory adaptation at 2 mi/hr, 0% grade. It then increases 2 METs every 2 minutes. This provides enough data to generate response curves for incremental heart rate, blood pressure, electrocardiographic responses, and rate of perceived exertion.

Baseline blood pressure and a resting electrocardiogram are taken before the start of the exercise test. We use a bipolar V5 lead along the long axis of the heart, an anterior V2 type lead, and an inferior lead such as AVF to monitor the exercise electrocardiogram. With this lead system almost 90% of electrocardiographic changes due to ischemia can be detected. During the testing, the oscilloscope is continuously monitored for dysrhythmias and other electrocardiographic changes. Determinations of blood pressure and heart rate are also recorded in the last half-minute of each stage and every minute during recovery until normal levels are reached (at least 5 to 9 minutes). More frequent measurements may be desirable in the presence of certain abnormalities.

At the end of the test the treadmill is slowed down for about 30 seconds. The patient should be placed in a supine position for the recovery period if exercise is abruptly interrupted or for diagnostic observations.[1] Ordinarily, if the test is done for other than diagnostic purposes, a cool-down walk is desirable.

Limiting Signs

While submaximal testing can be useful, we prefer maximal or symptom-limited testing because the sensitivity is increased and functional capacity can be estimated more accurately.

Exercise capacity is dependent upon the efficiency of the respiratory and cardiovascular systems, adequacy of blood components, and the cellular enzymes that help the body utilize oxygen during exercise.

The capacity of the heart to pump the blood to all bodily systems is the most important factor in the oxygen transport. Pulmonary factors do not limit exercise performance unless significant pulmonary disease is present. Under normal conditions and at sea level, arterial blood leaving the heart is approximately 97% saturated with oxygen and therefore most of the limitations to exercise performance depend on the capacity of the heart and circulation and on cellular function.[5]

In healthy individuals under normal conditions, exercise is limited by muscular fatigue when maximum oxygen uptake is reached. At this point, maximum cardiac output is reached as well.

During the testing, the physician conducting the test must maintain close visual observation and verbal communication with the patient in order to recognize early signs or symptoms and to make sure that the patient does not minimize any discomfort.

With symptom-limited testing, the following symptoms relating to the cardiovascular system are indications for terminating the test[6]:

1. *Angina pectoris* Well-known characteristics of this symptom are not only its localization but also its presentation with increasing effort and its resolution by rest or nitroglycerine. However, the nitroglycerine response is less specific than was previously thought; pain from spasm of the esophagus also is relieved by nitroglycerine.

2. *Dyspnea* When its presentation is not related to pulmonary disease, it is an expression of cardiac failure, especially if it is accompanied by S4 and congestive rales.

3. *Blood pressure* A drop in systolic blood pressure or a lack of increase during exercise can be a critical sign of cardiac pump failure, especially if it is accompanied by pallor, cold perspiration, ataxia, or any other sign of low cardiac output. Blood pressure elevation to 250 mmHg systolic or 130 mmHg diastolic is also a limiting factor. A slight drop in blood pressure after the end of the test without any other evidence of hemodynamic failure is not an infrequent finding in normal individuals.

4. *Claudication* Pain in the lower extremities is another limiting sign caused by peripheral artery insufficiency.

5. *Electrocardiographic signs* Significant arrhythmias include ventricular tachycardia, polymorphic extrasystoles, tachy- or brady-arrhythmias, and AV block. ST segment depression greater than 3 mm (.3 mv) and ST segment elevation as an expression of subepicardial ischemia are also reasons for suspending the test.

Interpretation of the Treadmill Test

The interpretation of the treadmill exercise test requires the analysis of the hemodynamic and the electrocardiographic responses to exercise as well as evaluation of the signs and symptoms of disease.

Traditionally, the treadmill exercise test has been used for the diagnosis of coronary heart disease. Therefore, the terms "normal" or "negative" and "positive" or "abnormal" have been used as synonyms. A positive test means that angina pectoris and/or ST segment depression occurred, suggesting coronary heart disease. However, in the treadmill test report it is preferable to describe the particular clinical or electrocardiographic responses that were considered diagnostically important. A "negative" test is not necessarily normal; "negative" usually means only that the patient completed the treadmill test without having angina pectoris or significant ST segment depression. But the patient could have had other noteworthy symptoms such as dyspnea or dizziness, or an arrhythmia or other electrocardiographic abnormality.

The significance of the heart rate, blood pressure, and electrocardiographic responses in interpreting the results will be discussed below.

Heart Rate Response

The increase in heart rate at the various stages as well as the maximum rate achieved are compared with the expected rates for men/women of the same age.

The heart rate increases with increasing workload. For men, it increases approximately 8 to 10 beats/min for each MET increase[7] and for women about 11 to 13 beats/min for each MET increase.[5] Heart rate response per MET is higher in sedentary than in trained individuals.[5]

Maximum heart rate response is inversely correlated with age. In healthy individuals this could be estimated by subtracting age from 220 (low estimate), or by subtracting half the age from 210 (high estimate). Thus for a 46-year-old man, the maximum predicted heart rate response is between 174 and 187. This estimate can be used as a guide but not as a predetermined end point for the exercise test since there is great variation in heart rate response. The standard deviation for maximal heart rate is approximately ± 12 beats/min.[6]

As mentioned above, there is normally a linear relationship between percent of maximal heart rate and percent of maximal oxygen uptake. VO_2 Max is achieved when the VO_2 does not increase with further increments in the intensity of exercise. This also is the point at which maximal heart rate is attained. For this reason, the heart rate can serve to monitor fitness progress. In clinical populations, the relationship between heart rate and oxygen uptake is not strictly linear, and the maximal heart rate may be overestimated by this method of calculation.[8]

Elevated heart rate response to exercise could be due to anemia, cardiac failure, metabolic disorders, anxiety or elevated sympathetic tone.

A low heart rate response could be due to the training effect, medication (especially beta blockers), or coronary insufficiency. Ellestad[9] called the inability to increase the heart rate during exercise "chronotropic incompetance" and recognized it as a sign of coronary insufficiency and a marker for future coronary events.

During the recovery period after the test, the heart rate returns to preexercise levels, but this takes more time in sedentary persons than in conditioned individuals.[7]

Blood Pressure Response

Systolic blood pressure increases linearly with increased levels of exercise. The average systolic blood pressure response is an increase of 7 to 10 mmHg for each MET increase in workload.[7] Diastolic blood pressure remains constant or decreases slightly during dynamic treadmill exercise. During bicycle ergometer exercise, diastolic blood pressure could increase due to the isometric component of the exercise.

Although elevations in blood pressure to 250 mmHg systolic or to 130 mmHg diastolic are indications to terminate the test, their actual significance is not clear. However, no change or a drop in systolic blood pressure with increasing exercise is a marker for increased risk for cardiovascular events especially for patients with preexisting coronary heart disease.[10]

In our experience, elevated levels or a surge in blood pressure during the warmup stage of exercise correlate with labile hypertension and hot reacting.[11] Elevated systolic blood pressure during recovery is a marker for future established hypertension.[12] Exercise-related blood pressure may be useful as a screening test in predicting the subsequent development of hypertension.

An increase in diastolic blood pressure during exercise can be an indication of left ventricular dysfunction in patients with coronary artery disease.

Electrocardiographic Abnormalities

Horizontal or down-sloping ST-T displacement of more than 0.1 mv below the resting isoelectric point for at least 80 milliseconds is the most accepted manifestation of exercise-induced myocardial ischemia.

Some conditions other than coronary insufficiency can result in false positive ST-T changes. The most important is left ventricular hypertrophy possibly accompanying valvular, congenital, or myocardial heart disease as well as hypertension. Certain drugs can cause exercise-induced repolarization abnormalities; digitalis is the most common of these. Other possible causes of an abnormal ECG response are anemia, electrolyte imbalance, vasoregulatory abnormalities, mitral valve prolapse, pericardial effusions, preexcitation syndromes (Wolff-Parkinson-White) and left bundle branch block.[10] Because meals and glucose ingestion can alter the ST-T segment and cause a false positive response, all exercise tests should be performed after a minimum of 4 hours of fasting.

Individuals with labile ST-T wave changes have an increased incidence of false positive ST segment depression with exercise. If hyperventilation produces ST segment changes or a reversal of the T wave, then abnormal ST segment depression must be interpreted with caution. The incidence of false positive ST segment responses to exercise is higher in women than in men. Indeed, the exercise test may be useful mainly as a prognostic test, not a diagnostic test, in women.[2]

Certain attributes of the ST segment contribute to the prognostic accuracy of the exercise test. Specificity for myocardial ischemia is increased the lower the workload, heart rate or double product at which ST depression occurs. Upsloping ST segments are less indicative of ischemia than flat or down-sloping ST segments. ST-T complexes that go through a phase of ST depression with a temporary downward-upward diphasic T-wave contour in the recovery period suggest more severe coronary artery disease than ST depression that resolves without developing diphasic T waves.[13]

In patients without evidence of necrosis on the electrocardiogram, the development of a septal Q wave in the V5 lead can be of great help in the diagnosis of ischemia. Significant ST segment depression without a Q wave at peak exercise is usually a true positive response for ischemia, yet ST segment depression at peak exercise with significant Q-wave voltage is suggestive of a false positive response.[14]

Another highly specific marker for ischemia is exercise-induced ST segment elevation; this rarely occurs in patients with normal resting electrocardiograms. Most of the time its presentation is associated with ventricular aneurysms in patients with previous anterior wall myocardial infarctions. (QS complexes in precordial leads.) Exercise-induced negative U waves have been associated with critical stenoses of the major coronary arteries, particularly the proximal left anterior descending coronary artery and the left main coronary artery.[17]

Patients with Prinzmetal angina tend to have ST segment elevation rather than ST segment depression. Waters et al[18] noted that on exercise testing these patients, one third had ST segment elevation, about one fourth showed ST segment depression, and in slightly less than one half, there were no ST segment abnormalities. They concluded that the exercise test could not define a high risk subgroup or predict the underlying coronary anatomy in variant angina. Others[19] surmise that the frequent false negative responses in these patients are due to the presence of a good coronary reserve or to a daily circadian variation in the tone of the coronary arteries.

Sensitivity and Specificity

Sensitivity is the ability of the exercise test to identify individuals with disease. It is expressed by the ratio of true positive responders to the total of true positives plus false negatives.

Specificity is the ability to identify individuals without disease. It is expressed as the ratio of true negatives to the total of true negatives plus false positives.

If the number of false negatives increases, the sensitivity decreases. If the number of false positives increases, the specificity decreases. With more stringent criteria for diagnosis, the sensitivity decreases and the specificity increases. If the number of leads used to monitor the electrocardiographic responses is increased, the sensitivity increases and the specificity decreases.[2] Using ST segment depression as the criterion for abnormality, the exercise test has been estimated to have a sensitivity of 50% and specificity of 90% for men on the average.[2] While the specificity for women is about the same, the sensitivity is much lower. Therefore, the predictive value of exercise testing is useful for men, particularly for symptomatic men, but only a negative test is meaningful for women.

Where clarification is required, exercise radionuclide studies or thallium-201 scans of the heart can be clinically important for evaluation of patients with known or suspected coronary artery disease. Radionuclide ventriculography provides quantitative measures of biventricular function and regional wall motion. Thallium-201 scans provide maps of regional myocardial perfusion.[15]

The sensitivity and specificity of thallium-201 myocardial imaging and radionuclide ventriculography for the detection of ischemic heart disease have been examined widely. Both techniques appear to be more sensitive than exercise electrocardiography and are more useful with patients having baseline electrocardiographic abnormalities due to cardiovascular drugs, left ventricular hypertrophy, or the presence of intraventricular conduction abnormalities.[15]

The specificity of exercise thallium-201 myocardial imaging is also better than that of exercise electrocardiography, approximately 85 to 90% versus 70 to 85%. The specificity of exercise radionuclide ventriculography may be considerably lower than that for exercise electrocardiography, depending on the population studied. Improvements in instrumentation and computer analyses of the data have enhanced both specificity and sensitivity of these techniques. However, they have many limitations including individual variations in both patients and observers.[15]

Thallium-201 imaging is particularly useful for differentiating reversible manifestations of ischemia from perfusion defects and for evaluating response to perfusion therapy. Radionuclide angiography is especially helpful in assessment of ventricular performance, both for diagnostic purposes and to evaluate therapy. Helpful guidelines for use of cardiac radionuclide imaging techniques have recently been published.[16]

Exercise Prescription

Purpose of Exercise

The role of intense and vigorous exercise in human health remains a controversial issue, although there is general agreement that moderate and regular aerobic exercise is an essential component of the healthy life style. Training consistently improves physical strength, efficiency, and capacity associated with increased cardiorespiratory performance. It increases the ability to deliver and utilize oxygen and improves muscular, neurological, pulmonary, metabolic, and hemodynamic functions. In some cases it has been found to increase the level of HDL in the blood and to be associated with lower blood pressure in mild hypertensives.[20] Potential behavioral benefits of regular exercise include reduction of anxiety and depression and improvement in confidence and self-esteem.[21]

For weight control, the combination of diet and exercise aids loss of fat and decreases loss of protein, compared to diet alone. It seems to reset the "set point" for basal metabolism at a higher rate so that weight loss is steadier and maintained longer in those who remain active. Exercise also tends to normalize the glucose metabolism, reducing the risk of diabetes, lowering insulin requirements, and dropping triglyceride blood levels.[22]

Contrary to common belief, increased activity does not necessarily increase the appetite. A study of caloric intake of workers having different activity levels showed that sedentary individuals ate more than those having moderate activity.[23] Furthermore, the body revs up the metabolic rate before exercise starts and keeps the rate up for hours afterward.[22] This results in a greater consumption of calories than would be expected just from the exercise activity alone. The physiological basis is believed to be increased stimulation of the sympathetic nervous system.

Preliminary Considerations

The attending physician should be familiar with appropriate medical evaluation and recommendations for initiating an exercise program for a variety of individuals. The contraindications for exercise training are the same as for exercise testing. Additionally special considerations are called for in certain cases of coronary patients and in the presence of other handicaps or disease.

As with any other treatment, the type of exercise and the "dosage" prescribed must be appropriate for the individual, sufficient to promote the training effect, while avoiding any potentially harmful side effects. A complete evaluation of the patient is needed in order to determine the correct dosage including the type, intensity, duration, frequency, and progression of physical activity. This evaluation is based on the exercise test, the patient's medical state, coronary risk profile, attitude toward exercise, motivation, lifestyle, climate and musculoskeletal stability.

Work Capacity

The treadmill test provides the most objective evaluation for establishing the exercise "dosage." However, graded exercise testing is not necessary for healthy adults under 30 years of age, or those 30 to 40 with low cardiovascular risk, unless their chosen physical activity is particularly strenuous. All cardiovascular patients and asymptomatic individuals who are over 40 years of age should have an exercise test before entering an exercise program.[1]

Determination of the work capacity of the individual must take into consideration the maximal work load completed on the treadmill, hemodynamic measurements such as blood pressure and heart rate as a function of exercise intensity, electrocardiographic responses before, during, and after exercise, and signs and symptoms of cardiovascular disease.

During progressive aerobic exercise, cardiac output and heart rate increase in direct proportion to the percentage of VO_2 max. Heart rate is the major determinant of cardiac output at work intensities above 50% of VO_2 max, so that a linear increase in heart rate provides qualitative evidence of increased cardiac output. In the absence of disease or drug effects, the heart rate is also linearly related to myocardial and body oxygen consumption. Therefore, when maximal heart rate is achieved in the treadmill test, maximal myocardial and body oxygen consumption are also achieved.

Figure 1 shows the difference in workloads achieved by two young individuals with different levels of fitness. The trained individual can achieve a workload of 10 METs with 160 beats/min, while the untrained one "needs" 200 beats/min to reach that workload. Because of the linear relationship between workload in METs and heart rate for a given individual, the heart rate can indicate the work being done by the individual; it is used to monitor the dynamic exercise intensity.

Type of Exercise

Physical activity involves two types of muscle contractions—isotonic or dynamic, and isometric or static. Isotonic or dynamic exercise is the usual repetitive or rhythmic contraction of large muscle groups

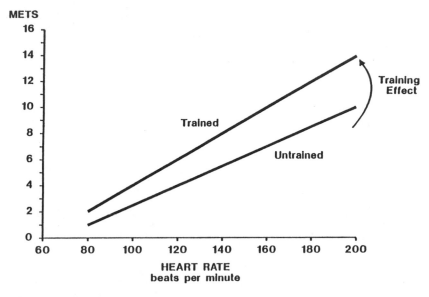

Figure 1: The trained individual achieves a given workload (METS) with less heart-beat "expense" than the untrained person.

associated with any nearly continuous motion of part of the body; it requires an increase in cardiac output, ventilation, and oxygen consumption. It is also called aerobic because it requires a continuous oxygen supply. Examples of dynamic exercise are walking, running, swimming, and bicycling.

Static or isometric exercise consists of sustained muscle contractions that produce little or no motion of the involved body part. It can overload the heart as it tends to raise the mean blood pressure without increasing cardiac output. For this reason, this type of exercise should be a minimal component in an exercise program for cardiac patients and hypertensives. Weight lifting is mainly an isometric exercise. As evidence of this, we have seen remarkable surges during the handgrip test of "hot reactors."

Regular isotonic exercise helps maintain strength by slowing the decrease in fiber size of type II (aerobic, fast-twitch) muscle fibers that occurs with aging and deconditioning.[5] In an aerobic training program, the isotonic contraction of large muscles should be the major component of exercise, and the isometric component should be minimized.

The exercise can be continuous, as with brisk walking, or intermittent, as in tennis or jog-walk programs. Continuous types of exercise achieve the target heart rate more quickly and sustain it for a longer time, but the intermittent types are often easier for less fit individuals and may also include a greater variety of enjoyable activities.

The stationary bicycle is widely used for physical training because it permits a good control of both workload and heart rate during exercising. It lends itself to home use as it takes up little space and permits the user to read or watch TV at the same time. The MET cost of bicycling depends on body weight.

Intensity

Studies have shown that healthy young individuals can develop and maintain cardiorespiratory fitness at an intensity of exercise that raises the heart rate to 130 or more beats/min, or that requires approximately 60% of maximum heart rate reserve. This threshold can fluctuate significantly, depending on levels of fitness, with lower levels in less fit persons and higher levels in well trained ones.[23] The higher intensity of training is associated with more frequent injuries, especially in those just starting an exercise program. If exercise is too intense (that is at too high a training heart rate) the exercise may become predominantly anaerobic. Therefore there are both maximal and minimal heart rates delineating the zone where the aerobic training effect is obtained. This training zone varies, as mentioned, with the level of fitness and of course with age, since the maximal heart rate response is inversely related to age. To obtain the training heart rate, the intensity of exercise should be between 50% and 85% of maximum heart rate reserve. Karvonen[24] developed a formula based on the maximum heart rate reserve which provides the range for the training heart rate (THR). It is calculated as follows:

THR = 50 to 85% × (Max HR − Resting HR) + Resting HR,

For example, if the maximal heart rate is 180 beats/min and the resting heart rate is 80 beats/min, the lower limit of the training zone will be 50% × (180 − 80) + 80 = 130 beats/min; and the upper limit will be 85% times (180 − 80) + 80 = 165 beats/min.

Young healthy individuals with better levels of fitness can train close to the maximal heart rate of the training zone. On the other hand, older individuals, those with low levels of fitness, and cardiac patients should train close to the lower limit of the training zone. Here are two examples illustrating this point.

The first case is a 20-year-old healthy man, physically active. He doesn't fit the criteria for doing a graded exercise test, so we calculate his maximal heart rate by subtracting his age from 220 for the low estimate. Then, using his resting heart rate, which is 70 beats/min, the training heart rate will equal 85%(200 − 70) + 70 = 180.5 beats/min.

The second case is a 60-year-old sedentary man with a previous myocardial infarction who decides to undergo an exercise program. A treadmill exercise test is necessary in this case, and the maximal heart rate he achieves without symptoms (angina or electrocardiographic signs of ischemia) will be used as the maximal heart rate in the formula. His maximal heart rate during the exercise test turns out to be 140 beats/min, and his resting heart rate is 70, so the lowest training heart rate will be:

$$50\%(140 - 70) + 70 = 105 \text{ beats/min.}$$

and that is the level at which he should train.

Duration of Training

Improvement in aerobic capacity is directly related to the duration of training. If the intensity is kept constant, exercise programs of shorter duration produce significantly less effect than do programs of longer duration. The duration of exercise training sessions can vary from 15 to 60 minutes and generally depends on the desired intensity. It has been demonstrated that exercise regimens of lower intensity but with a longer duration produce improvements similar to those of the higher intensities and shorter duration if the total kilocaloric expenditures are approximately equal for both programs.[5] As long as the intensity is above the minimal threshold level and a certain amount of total work is completed in an exercise session, the manner in which the end result is accomplished can vary. In general, an optimal rate of improvement in fitness is attained by expending approximately 300 Cal per exercise session. However, individuals who have previously been very sedentary should work up to this level gradually, starting at perhaps only 100 to 200 Cal per session.

The treadmill test indicates the heart rate of the patient at various work loads (METS). Since 1 MET requires 1 Cal/kg.hr, we can calculate the patient's caloric expenditure per MET level and then determine the proper duration of the training session, based on the caloric expenditure for a given heart rate. If an individual's training heart rate of 140 beats/min corresponds to 5 METS on the treadmill test, the caloric expenditure for that heart rate will be 5 Cal/kg/hr. If the individual weighs 70 kg (154 lb) the caloric cost will be 350 Cal/hr or 5.8 Cal/min. If a total caloric expenditure of 200 Cal is required, the duration of the training session should be approximately 35 minutes (200/5.8 = 34.48). Exercise programs with high intensity and short duration are more suitable for young healthy people with good levels of fitness. For cardiac patients or persons with low levels of fitness, exercise training sessions with low intensity and longer duration can be designed for the desired caloric expenditure (200–400 Cal).

Frequency

In general the ideal frequency has been found to be once a day, three to five times a week. If exercise sessions are too widely spaced, gains in physical conditioning may be lost. Exercise sessions less than three times per week produce minimal cardiorespiratory improvements, but the frequency may vary as a function of intensity and duration. If duration and intensity are very low, the frequency can be increased to twice a day. Frequency also depends on the mode of exercise and the individual's needs. Sessions three times a week with at least 20 minutes at the training heart rate are suitable for most individuals.

Tables 1 and 2 are examples of exercise prescriptions, one for a healthy middle-aged individual, the other for an older patient who has had a myocardial infarction.

Structure of the Training Program

The most beneficial schedule for beginners of average fitness is a program of 3 days per week, about 30 minutes per session of aerobic exercise at an intensity that is perceived as neither very easy nor really hard. (See Table 3, Subjective ratings of perceived exertion). This will correspond to a heart rate of about 110 to 140 beats/min. Longer or more frequent sessions increase the risk of injury. Allowing at least one day between sessions gives the individual time to get over the fatigue or achiness of the previous session. Exercising twice a week for longer periods provides about the same conditioning, but is not effective for weight loss.[5]

For healthy individuals, the exercise should be in the form of enjoyable activities that can become a regular habit. Swimming, fast walking,

Table 1
Exercise Prescription

Name:
Cardiovascular Diagnosis: None
Other Diagnosis: None
Age: 45
Medication: None
Weight: 70 Kg (154 lb)

Treadmill Test Results

Stage	Time min	Speed mph	Grade %	METS	VO₂ ml/kg/m	Cal/h/ Kg	HR bpm	BP mmHg	RPE Borg	ECG ST	Angina
0				1	3.5	1	85	112/76			
1	2	2.0	0	2	7	2	99	114/84	10		
2	2	3.0	2.5	4	14	4	107	122/78	11		
3	2	3.0	7.5	6	21	6	118	134/78	12		
4	2	3.4	10	8	28	8	138	150/78	14		
5	2	3.4	14	10	35	10	161	168/86	17		
6	2	3.7	16	12	42	12	175	180/85	19		

PRESCRIPTION

Intensity: METS—From 8 to 10, or VO₂ From 28 to 35 ml/kg/min
Training Heart Rate—From 130 to 162 bpm
RPE—From 13 to 16
Duration: 30 min or From 8 to 10 Cal/Kg/h (Average = 9), or 300 Cal
Frequency: 3 times per week
Progression: Start with 5 minute warm-up, 10 minute training and 5 minute cool-down. Increase training time 5 minutes each week until training time equals 30 minutes.
Type-mode: Walking—running—walking

Table 2
Exercise Prescription

Name: Age: 56
Cardiovascular Diagnosis: Myocardial infarction
Other diagnosis: None

Medication: Diltiazem
Weight: 80 Kg (176 lb)

Treadmill Test Results

Stage	Time min	Speed mph	Grade %	METS	VO_2 ml/kg/m	Cal/h/Kg	HR bpm	BP mmHg	RPE Borg	ECG ST	Angina
0				1	3.5	1	80	140/90			
1	2	2.0	0	2	7	2	107	150/90	10		
2	2	3.0	2.5	4	14	4	115	170/90	12		
3	2	3.0	7.5	6	21	6	135	190/90	15		
4	2	3.4	10.0	8	28	8	150	210/90	17	2mm	+

PRESCRIPTION
Intensity: METS—From 2 to 5, or VO_2 From 7 to 17 ml/kg/min
              Training Heart Rate—From 107 to 127 bpm
              RPE—From 10 to 13
Duration: 43 min or From 2 to 5 Cal/Kg/h (Average = 3.5), or 200 Cal
Frequency: 3 times per week
Progression: Start with 5 minutes of warmup, 10 minutes of walking, and a 5 minute cool-down. Increase training time 5 minutes each week
              until training time equals 43 minutes.
Type-mode: Walking

dancing, bicycling, etc. are all good aerobic exercises. The activities can be varied, and for those who prefer a daily exercise time, lower level activities can alternate with the more vigorous ones. For a well rounded program, strength and flexibility exercises should be included as well as endurance training.

All training sessions should include the following periods: the warm-up, the training zone exercise, and the cool-down. The 30-minute routine might include 10 minutes of warm-up, 15 minutes of continuous vigorous activity, and 5 minutes of cool-down. For beginners, the warm-up and cool-down periods may be longer.

The importance of the warm-up and cool-down should be stressed. Most people understand the purpose of the warm-up: limbering up exercises to loosen and warm up the muscles and joints, like warming up the engine on the car on a cold day to permit all the parts to be lubricated and in good running order before being stressed. The need for the cool-down may not be so obvious, as cars can be stopped and turned off abruptly after a trip. Of course, the human engine isn't turned off after exercise. During vigorous activity such as running, for instance, blood vessels in the legs expand to maximize the oxygen

Table 3
Borg's Scale
Ratings of Perceived Exertion (RPE)

RPE	Approx Heart Rate (bpm)
6	60
7 Very, very easy	70
8	80
9 Very easy	90
10	100
11 Fairly easy	110
12	120
13 Somewhat hard	130
14	140
15 Hard	150
16	160
17 Very hard	170
18	180
19 Very, very hard	190
20	200

reaching the working muscles. The action of the muscles helps push the blood through the veins back to the heart. If the activity is abruptly stopped, the extra blood will be pooled in the legs instead of being pushed up to the heart which is still beating fast and working hard. As a result, the volume of blood reaching the heart will suddenly be diminished, and there will be inadequate forward flow to the brain (causing light-headedness) or underfilling of the coronary arteries (which can lead to arrhythmias or myocardial ischemia). During the cool-down, the arteries in the legs will gradually constrict, and the volume of blood sent back to the heart can be redistributed; meanwhile, the heart beat slows down, diminishing myocardial requirements.[5]

The Warm-up

Warm-ups are low intensity repetitions that gradually adjust the body's temperature, respiration, and circulation to the increasing activity. It generally includes stretching exercises for the lower back, hamstring and calf muscles to prevent and/or reduce risk of injury. Moderate walking or flexibility exercises are also suitable. The warm-up period usually lasts 5 to 10 minutes.

Training-Zone Exercise

The major portion of the exercise session is the aerobic exercise at the target or training heart rate. This may be in the form of low intensity steady-state training or high intensity interval training. Whether the endurance conditioning is continuous or discontinuous depends on the individual's age, health status, functional capacity, or level of fitness, as well as exercise interests, time available, equipment, facilities, and objectives. Duration of the aerobic exercise in the training zone can vary from 15 to 60 minutes and can include walking, cycling, running, sports, etc.

The Cool-Down

The cool-down period consists of exercise of diminishing intensity, for example, slower walking, stretching exercises, and muscle relaxation. It should be continued until the heart rate is no longer rapidly decreasing, generally about 5 minutes.

Progression

The rate of progress is related to the intensity, duration, and frequency of exercise sessions, which in turn depend on the individual health status and physical fitness. For cardiac patients, periodic graded exercise tests can be used to monitor improvement and to indicate when an individual can safely increase the level of exercise—by changing intensity, duration, caloric expenditure, or type of exercise. The adjustment in healthy individuals could be based simply on the observed exercise performance. In most cases, cardiac patients can achieve a satisfactory level of cardiorespiratory fitness after about six months in a supervised exercise program. At this point, further improvements may be minimal, and the main goal is to establish a maintenance program that the patient can continue without supervision in order to sustain the improvement.

Fitness effects are most notable in those who begin training from a low level of fitness. Even minimal increases in activity as low as 5 minutes per day can increase the VO_2 max and flexibility of the very unfit. Longer, more intense training would be needed to improve those with greater fitness. It has been found that expenditures of more than 600 calories per day add little to one's fitness and increase the risk of injury.[3]

It takes less effort to maintain fitness than to attain it. Unfortunately, if it is not maintained, it again requires marked effort to regain what has been lost—and the higher the level to be regained the more effort required. Aerobic capacity drops significantly after 1 or 2 weeks of detraining and continues to drop if exercise is not resumed. In one experiment, trained and untrained individuals were given 20 days of bed rest followed by 60 days of exercise training.[25] Besides demonstrating the deconditioning effects of prolonged bed rest, this study showed that the trained individuals required 40 days of training to achieve their pre-resting fitness level, but the untrained individuals achieved their pre-resting level in only 14 days.

Dangers and Cautions

One of the potentially fatal mistakes that is often made is the return to the same level of physical activity following a period of illness or layoff. A good rule of thumb offered by Dehn and Mullins[26] is to decrease one work level for every workout missed and then gradually increase the level at each session.

While treadmill testing is recommended for persons at risk of cardiovascular disease, it should be recognized that a good result may give a false sense of assurance. Each person should "listen" to his/her own body and be aware of any changes or discomforts.

Patients should be informed of signs that indicate they should stop an exercise or skip the exercise session. These include palpitations, fluttering, arrhythmias or other abnormal heart activity; pain or pressure in the chest, arm or throat occurring while exercising or soon thereafter; dizziness, confusion, cold sweat or cyanosis. Exercise also should not be undertaken during an illness especially if there is fever.[27]

A recent conference at UCLA reviewed the literature on exercise and concluded that while joggers had a greater risk of death during or just after exercise than when they were at rest, their overall morbidity and mortality from cardiovascular disease were lower that those for sedentary persons.[20] Those most at risk for exercise-related death were men who were not used to strenuous exercise before they indulged in vigorous activity. Furthermore, they point out that the risk of death from physical activity is comparable to the risk posed by complications of medication and medical procedures.

Among young athletes dying during or just after exercise, the main cause is hypertrophic cardiomyopathy, usually of genetic origin. This indicates the great importance of taking a good family history before admitting persons, especially young persons, to strenuous sports activities.

On the positive side, Paffenberger's ongoing study of male college graduates indicates that those who continue to be physically active, whether or not they were athletes in college, tend to be healthier. The prognosis correlated with the amount of exercise up to the consumption of about 2000 calories per week.[28]

Jogging, particularly marathon running, has been popularized as a method almost capable of immunizing against cardiovascular disease. However, there are various other risks associated with this sport. These include heat stroke, anaphylactic reactions, stress fractures and other musculoskeletal injuries, dog bites, and being struck by objects including cars.

Lately there has been concern about excessive jogging which can lead to addiction, anorexia, metabolic changes such as potassium and magnesium deficiency, endocrine changes, amenorrhea, decreased testosterone, etc. Also the sudden interest and shift from jogging to cycling is possibly due in part to orthopedic complications precluding jogging. Clearly it is unfortunate to lose cardiovascular fitness because of such complications, yet in my experience, this is not uncommon. Walking is a lifetime aerobic activity that can be pursued by 97% of the population until the day they die. It is a conditioning activity that is ubiquitous, social, applicable in a variety of settings, and no special equipment is required.

Some simple precautions can reduce the hazards of running or walking. In general, do not run after dark; run against traffic; run in single file; and wear proper footwear and clothing suitable to the weather. To prevent anaphylactic reactions, persons with known food allergies should not eat anything they are allergic to (especially shellfish and celery) for two hours before strenuous exercise[29].

Patients should be instructed to take warm rather than hot showers after exercising and not to use saunas at such times. The heat causes a marked reduction in peripheral resistance and can lead to hypovolemia, with fainting, arrythmias, or worse.

Both extremes of heat and cold add to the stress on the body during exercise and should be avoided by cardiac patients. Even swimming in cold water can be a hazard. Anyone exercising in hot conditions should dress suitably and drink plenty of fluids before, during, and after the exercise if they are perspiring profusely. For cold weather it is best to wear layers of clothing so that some can be removed when the individual has warmed up. Sweat-soaked clothing can lead to rapid chilling. It is also important to wear a head covering such as a stocking cap since there is a large heat loss from the head.

Vigorous exercise may be too hazardous for cardiac patients in certain conditions, but those judged able to undergo rehabilitative exercise will probably benefit. Exercise can be an important therapy. Like any prescription, one must be assured that it is safe, effective, and prudent for the patient in question.

Although secondary intervention in coronary heart disease has not proved statistically to reduce mortality, clear trends toward increased survival have been found. Exercise does not seem to worsen prognosis and may be shown to enhance it when done sensibily, in moderation.

References

1. American College of Sports Medicine. Guidelines for Graded Exercise Testing and Exercise Prescription. Lea & Febiger, Philadelphia, 1980.

2. Schlant RC, Blomqvist CG, Brandenburg RO, et al. Guidelines for exercise testing: A report of the American College of Cardiology/American Heart Association Task Force on Assessment of Cardiovascular Procedures (Subcommittee on Exercise Testing). JACC 8:725–738, 1986.
3. Sharkey BJ. Physiology of Fitness. Human Kinetics Publishers, Inc., Champaign, Ill., 1984. Appendix A, Muscles, energy, and oxygen. pp 235–254.
4. Fletcher GF, Mikolich JR. The exercise prescription. In: Fletcher GF (ed). Exercise in the Practice of Medicine. Futura Publishing Company, Inc., Mount Kisco, N.Y., 1982. pp 77–102.
5. Pollock, ML, Wilmore JH, Fox SM III. Exercise in Health and Disease. W.B. Saunders Company, Philadelphia, 1984.
6. Froelicher VF. Exercise Testing and Training. Year Book Medical Publishers, Inc., Chicago, 1983.
7. American Heart Association: Exercise Testing and Training of Individuals with Heart Disease or at High Risk for its Development: A Handbook for Physicians. Dallas, American Heart Association, 1975.
8. Dressendorfer RH, Smith JL. Predictive accuracy of the maximum heart rate reserve method for estimating aerobic training intensity in early cardiac rehabilitation. J Cardiac Rehabil 4:484–489, 1984.
9. Ellestad MH, Wan MKC. Predictive implications of stress testing: Followup of 2700 subjects after maximal treadmill stress test. Circulation 51:363, 1975.
10. Schlant RC, Blomqvist CG, Brandenburg RO, et al. Guidelines for exercise testing, a report of the American College of Cardiology/American Heart Association Task Force on Assessment of Cardiovascular Procedures (Subcommittee on exercise testing). J Am Coll Cardiol 8:725–738, 1986.
11. Ruddel H, McKinney ME, Buell JC, et al. Low work load during physical stress testing is mental stress testing. In: Lollgen H, Mellerowicz H (eds). Progress in Ergometry: Quality Control and Test Criteria. Soringer-Verlag, Berlin, 1984. pp 222–228.
12. Davidoff R, Schamroth CL, Goldman AP, et al. Postexercise blood pressure as a predictor of hypertension. Aviat Space Environ Med 53:591–594, 1982.
13. Sheffield LT. Another perfect treadmill test? N Engl J Med 313:633–635, 1985.
14. Morales Ballejo HM, Greenberg PS, Ellestad MH, et al. The septal Q wave in exercise testing: angiographic correlation. Am J Cardiol 48:247–251, 1981.
15. Pitt B, Kalff V, Rabinovitch M, et al. Impact of radionuclide techniques on evaluation of patients with ischemic heart disease. J Am Coll Cardiol 1:63–72, 1983.
16. O'Rourke RA, Chatterjee K, Dodge HT, et al. Guidelines for clinical use of cardiac radionuclide imaging, December 1986, a report of the American College of Cardiology/American Heart Association Task Force on Assessment of Cardiovascular Procedures (Subcommittee on Nuclear Imaging). J Am Coll Cardiol 8:1471–1483, 1986.
17. Gerson MC, Phillips JF, Morris SN, et al. Exercise-induced U-wave inversion as a marker of stenosis of the left anterior descending coronary artery. Circulation 60:1014–1020, 1979.

18. Waters DD, Szlachcic J, Bourassa MG, et al. Exercise testing in patients with variant angina: results, correlation with clinical and angiographic features and prognostic significance. Circulation 65:265–74, 1982.
19. Carboni GP, Celli P, D'Ermo M, et al. Combined cardiac cinefluoroscopy, exercise testing, and ambulatory ST-segment monitoring in the diagnosis of CAD: a report of 106 symptomatic patients. J Cardiol 9(1):91–101, 1985.
20. Bairey CN. Exercise and coronary artery disease—What should we be recommending to our patients (and ourselves)?—Medical Staff Conference, University of California, San Francisco. West J Med 144:205–211, 1986.
21. Sime WE. Psychological benefits of exercise training in the healthy individual. In: Matarazzo JD, Weiss SM, Herd JA, Miller NE, Weiss SM (eds). Behavioral Health, John Wiley & Sons, New York, 1984. pp 488–508.
22. Donahoe CP Jr, Lin DH, Kirschenbaum DS, et al. Metabolic consequences of dieting and exercise in the treatment of obesity. J Consulting and Clin Psychol 52:827–836, 1984.
23. Guidelines for Exercise Testing and Prescription, 3rd edition. Lea & Febiger, Philadelphia, 1986, p 34.
24. Karvonen M, Kentala K, Musta O. The effects of training heart rate: a longitudinal study. Ann Med Exptl Biol Fenn 35:307–315, 1957. (Cited by Pollock, p 252.)
25. Saltin B, Blomqvist G, Mitchell JH, et al. Response to exercise after bedrest and after training. Circulation 38(Suppl 7):VII-1—VII-18, 1968.
26. Dehn MM, Mullins CB. Physiologic effects and importance of exercise in patients with coronary artery disease. Cardiovasc Med 2:365–387, 1977.
27. Zohman LR. Beyond Diet . . . Exercise Your Way to Fitness and Heart Health. Mazola Products, Best Foods, Englewood Cliffs, NJ 1974. (Cited by Pollock et al. p 379.)
28. Paffenberger RS Jr, Hyde RT, Wing AL. A natural history of athleticism and cardiovascular health. JAMA 252:491–495, 1984.
29. Kidd JM III, Cohen SH, Sosman AJ, et al. Food-dependent exercise-induced anaphylaxis. J Allergy Clin Immunol 71:407–411, 1983.

Chapter 10

Ambulatory Monitoring

Robert S. Eliot
Gregory A. Harshfield

The Need for Ambulatory Measurement

It was recognized over 40 years ago that traditional casual blood pressure measurements obtained in a physician's office are not truly representative of an individual's "usual" blood pressure.[1] The development of both an ambulatory intra-arterial blood pressure recorder[2] as well as a semiautomatic noninvasive ambulatory blood pressure recorder[3] emphasized the point, demonstrating the tremendous variability in blood pressure throughout the day. The clinical and research utility of these recorders was limited, however, because of the potential hazards in the case of the invasive device and the participation of the subject which was required in the case of the noninvasive device.[4] The introduction of fully automated, noninvasive blood pressure recorders has overcome these problems, opening up the potential for exciting new opportunities. Ambulatory ECG monitoring combined with the blood pressure measurements add to the usefulness of the devices.

Ambulatory Blood Pressure Measurement

Predictive Power

Devereux et al.[5] and others[6] found that ambulatory monitoring has prognostic significance in that those with higher average 24-hour blood

From: Eliot, RS: *Stress and the Heart: Mechanisms, Measurements and Management.* Mount Kisco, NY, Futura Publishing Company, Inc., © 1988.

pressures were more apt to develop established hypertension and left ventricular hypertrophy. Perloff et al.[7] found that those having higher blood pressure at home or work than would be predicted from office casual blood pressures are most at risk for both fatal and nonfatal cardiovascular events. Even elevated pressures in the doctor's office do not correlate well with 24-hour pressures. Thus office blood pressure has little prognostic or therapeutic reliability.

Clinical Utility

The principal uses for ambulatory blood pressure measurement are to identify hypertensives and to determine the effectiveness of therapy. Since clinic measurements of blood pressure can be misleading, particularly in patients who are apprehensive in the doctor's office, Harshfield recommends 24-hour monitoring before treatment is initiated, especially for borderline hypertensives. Of course, retaking of the blood pressure several times over a period of a month may be a cheaper method of identifying those with "white coat" hypertension. Hot reactors, who may have a higher blood pressure at work than in the doctor's office, can be identified with a mental stress test. The object in any case is to avoid subjecting persons not needing treatment (average diastolic 85 mmHg or less) to long-term medication of questionable value or the psychological impact of being labeled as hypertensive.

The mental stress tests we use have proved to correlate well with ambulatory monitoring,[8] both for revealing tendencies to have spikes of hypertension throughout the day (hot reacting) and for indicating mean waking blood pressure, the blood pressure that is most predictive of future target organ damage.

The average blood pressure over 24 hours determined by ambulatory measurement varies more than the blood pressure obtained during stress testing.[8] Therefore, to observe therapeutic effects, the stress blood pressure determination is more useful than ambulatory measurements.

Blood Pressure Monitors

There are currently five noninvasive ambulatory blood pressure recorders on the market. The oldest system is the Remler system. This system has the disadvantages of high cost as well as the necessity of active patient involvement in the blood pressure determination. It has the advantage of recording Karotkoff sounds, allowing for accurate data rejection.[9]

The second system is the Del Mar Avionics Ambulatory Blood Pressureometer II and ECG recorder. This system has the disadvantage of size (requiring the patient to wear two devices) and cost (requiring the purchase of two instruments and a scanner) but has the advantage of providing the physician with simultaneous records of blood pressure, heart rate, and ECG. In addition, it is easy to calibrate, stores the blood pressure determinations (allowing for editing by the human observer), and is based on the reliable ausculatory technique of blood pressure determination. Harshfield et al.,[10,11] and others[12,13] have performed extensive validation studies on the unit and found good agreement in approximately 80% of cases when auscultatory blood pressure measurements were taken by a trained observer with a mercury column and stethoscope while intra-arterial measurements were obtained simultaneously during cardiac catheterization.

For example, in Harshfield's validation study comparing the automated readings with auscultatory readings in 30 subjects, the correlation across subjects was 0.99 for systolic pressure and 0.94 for diastolic pressure with correlations for individual subjects ranging from 0.64 to 0.97 for systolic and 0.50 to 0.91 for diastolic pressure. Correlations with intra-arterial pressures on 10 subjects were 0.98 for both systolic and diastolic pressure.

The third device on the market is the Del Mar Avionics Pressurometer III, which provides both heart rate and blood pressure in a single unit. The unit operates exactly like the P II.

Another device, the Spacelabs recorder,[14] has the advantage of small size, but has two serious disadvantages: It is difficult, if not impossible, to calibrate, and it relies primarily on the oscillometric technique, which is not the most reliable.

The final unit is the Oxford Instruments device for which there are no reported validation or reliability studies as yet.

Procedures

Harshfield's group uses the following procedure. Prior to fitting the recorder on the patient, they obtain three consecutive blood pressure readings in the nondominant arm in each of the following conditions: sitting, standing, and reclining. A comparison of these readings with readings obtained later under comparable conditions during calibration/reactivity testing provides an index of the effect on blood pressure of the stress of wearing the recorder.

The subject is then seated in a comfortable chair and allowed to relax while the entire procedure is explained in detail.

Nine steps are involved in hookup.

1. The chest area is shaved and cleaned with alcohol for the placement of three ECG electrodes.
2. The ECG snap leads are connected to the electrodes and taped on to ensure that they will not become disconnected.
3. The brachial artery is examined in the antecubital fossa to determine the point at which the artery comes closest to the skin and maximal pulsation is felt.
4. A red dot is placed at the point determined in step 3.
5. The pressure transducer is placed over the artery such that the red dot lies directly beneath the center of the transducer.
6. The cuff is wrapped around the arm with the bladder entirely covering the transducer.
7. The leads are all connected to the blood pressure unit.
8. The P4 is also connected to a mercury column.
9. The P4 is set to the test mode which allows the technician to control the cuff deflation rate.

Blood pressure readings throughout the calibration and reactivity testing procedures are obtained simultaneously on the same arm by the P4 recorder and by a trained human observer, with the recorder inflating the cuff and the technician deflating the cuff. Three readings are obtained at one minute intervals during each of the following conditions: sitting, standing, reclining, mental arithmetic, isometric handgrip, and walking in place. The subjects are allowed a two-minute rest period following mental arithmetic, isometric handgrip, and walking in place. The subjects are asked to rate the physical and psychological demands of the latter three tests on a scale of 1 to 10.

These calibration/reactivity procedures serve several purposes. First, the physical and psychological demands of the different procedures test both the functioning of the recorders and the subject's reactivity with regard to physical and psychological tests. Also the different activities provide anchor points for comparison by which the subjects rate the physical and psychological demands of activities experienced throughout the ambulatory monitoring period.

The subjects are given a diary in which to record information for each blood pressure determination: time, blood pressure, location (work/home/sleep/ etc.), position (sitting, standing, reclining), activity (eating, walking, etc.), degree of physical exertion (on a scale of 1 to 10 based on the anchor points), and degree of mental exertion (on a scale of 1 to 10 based on the anchor points). Generally the timer is set to obtain readings at 15-minute intervals during the day and 30-minute intervals at night. The subjects are told to carry out their usual activities and return the following morning at which time the calibration procedure is repeated.

In addition the subjects are requested to obtain three readings at home during each of the same conditions as in the calibration procedure. This provides the blood pressure information without the potentially confounding influence of the laboratory environment. These readings also are important in comparing activity demands. Evaluations and adjustments can be made for each blood pressure reading to equate blood pressure information either across individuals or for the same individual across time.

The blood pressure and heart rate data are stored on magnetic tape, and when played back each reading is checked for validity. Readings are considered to be acceptable if the systolic pressure is at least 130% of the diastolic. Acceptable readings are then categorized according to the patient's activities.

ECG (Holter) Monitoring

Clinical Utility

Indications for ambulatory ECG monitoring[15] are as follows:

1. To reveal the circumstances leading to abnormalities such as episodic palpitation, light-headedness, dizziness, near and true syncope, and chest pain for purposes of diagnosis and evaluation.
2. To show cardiac arrhythmias for diagnosis or verification of control, or for prognosis in patients with structural heart disease.
3. To diagnose or show changes in frequency of symptomatic or asymptomatic myocardial ischemia (ST-segment shifts).
4. Evaluation of pacemaker function.
5. To monitor sleep.
6. To check the safety of new activities and rehabilitative exercise for a patient at risk.

Types of Monitors

Nowadays the recorders are small and light. They generally record from two ECG leads (usually modified V1 and V5) onto reel-to-reel or cassette tape. Some new systems can be programmed to monitor the occurrence of selective events identified by computer algorithm and/or patient trigger.[15] A three-channel system known as COMPAS is being used in Israel to detect premature ventricular contractions (PVC) as well as for differentiating arrhythmias and evaluating treatment.[16] Ohio State's University Hospitals even have a tiny device that patients can carry indefinitely, holding it to the chest when they feel the onset of a cardiac disturbance. The ECG results are then recorded over the telephone at the hospital.[17]

Tzivoni et al.[18] found that the two-lead Holter monitor was reliable for detecting ischemia, with similar sensitivity and specificity as in 12-lead stress tests. They used a V3-V5-like lead combination. While most ischemic changes were noted on the V5 lead, about 10% of their patients had ST-segment depression confined to V3. They believe the poor showing of early Holter monitors resulted mainly from their having only one lead. However, Tzivoni cautions that the capability of any Holter system should be validated by performing exercise tests on patients with normal and abnormal responses and recording ECG on both the 12-lead and Holter systems.

Some investigators have felt that the low-frequency response in Holter monitors was inadequate for detection of ST-segment abnormalities. Lambert et al.[19] have concluded from their study that ECG recording equipment does not require extended low-frequency range (such as that found in FM systems) to accurately reproduce these abnormalities.

ECG lead V1 is useful for identification of bundle branch block, differentiation of premature atrial contractions from premature ventricular beats, and separating supraventricular tachycardia with aberration from ventricular tachycardia.[15]

The playback scanners in use can replay the whole tape at 60 to 240 times real-time speed or select sample portions. They can be viewed on a screen or printed. Computer assistance enables them to select arrhythmic portions and even print summary graphs of such things as number of abnormal beats versus time.[15]

Interpretation

Detailed interpretation is beyond the scope of this discussion. The basic steps are as follows:[15]

1. Determine the basic ECG rhythm.
2. Determine the type, frequency, and time of occurrence of dysrhythmias, and other abnormalities.
3. Note the precise time of occurrence of clinically significant events and the patient's symptoms.
4. Determine the prognostic significance of the abnormalities found and the treatment, where required.

References

1. Ayman D, Goldshine AD. Blood pressure determinations by patients with essential hypertension I. The difference between clinic and home readings before treatment. Am J Med Sci 200:465–474, 1940.
2. Bevan AT, Honour AJ, Stott FD. Direct arterial pressure recording in unrestricted man. Clin Sci 36:329–344, 1969.
3. Sokolow M, Werdegar D, Keim HK, et al. Relationship between level of blood pressure measured casually and by portable records and severity of complications in essential hypertension. Circulation 34:279–298, 1966.
4. Pickering TG, Harshfield GA, Devereux RB, et al. What is the role of ambulatory blood pressure monitoring in the management of hypertensive patients? Hypertension 7:171–177, 1985.
5. Devereux RB, Pickering TG, Harshfield GA, et al. Left ventricular hypertrophy in patients with hypertension: importance of blood pressure response to regularly recurring stress. Circulation 68:470–476, 1983.
6. Mann S, Millar-Craig MW, Raftery EB. Superiority of 24-hour measurement of blood pressure over clinic values in determining prognosis in hypertension. Clin Exp Hypertens 7[A]:279–282, 1985.
7. Perloff D, Sokolow M, Cowan R. The prognostic value of ambulatory blood pressures. JAMA 249:2792–2798, 1983.
8. McKinney ME, Miner MH, Ruddel H, et al. The standardized mental stress protocol: test-retest reliability and comparison with ambulatory blood pressure monitoring. Psychophysiology 22:453–463, 1985.
9. Waeber B, des Combes DJ, Porchet M, et al. Accuracy, reproducibility, and usefulness of ambulatory blood pressure recording obtained with the Remler system. In: Weber MA, Drayer JIM (eds). Ambulatory Blood Pressure Monitoring. Steinkopff-Verlag Darmstadt 1984, pp 65–69.
10. Harshfield GA, Pickering TG, Laragh JH. A validation study of the Del Mar Avionics ambulatory blood pressure system. Ambulatory Electrocardiogr 1:7–12, 1979.
11. Harshfield GA, Pickering TG, Blank S, et al. Ambulatory blood pressure monitoring: records, applications, and analysis. In: Weber MA, Drayer JIM (eds). Ambulatory Blood Pressure Monitoring. Steinhopff-Verlag, Dannstadt 1984, pp 1–7.
12. Kennedy JL, Padgett NE, Horan MJ. Performance reliability of the Del Mar Avionics ambulatory blood pressure instrument in clinical use. Ambulatory Electrocardiogr 4:13–17, 1979.

13. Ward A, Hanson P. Accuracy and reproducibility of ambulatory blood pressure recorder measurements during rest and exercise. In: Weber MA, Drayer JIM (eds). Ambulatory Blood Pressure Monitoring. Steinhopff-Verlag, Dannstadt 1984, pp 51–56.
14. Dembroski TM, MacDougall JM. Validation of the Vita-Stat automated noninvasive ambulatory blood pressure recording device. In: Herd JA, Gotto AM, Kaufman PC, Weiss SM (eds). Cardiovascular Instrumentation: Application of New Technology to Biobehavioral Research. NIH Publication, No. 84-1654, 1984, pp 55–78.
15. Gessman LJ. Ambulatory Electrocardiography. Primary Cardiology 12(3):156–179, 1986.
16. Behar S, Ram GM, Neufeld HN. Real-time ambulatory detection of cardiac arrhythmias. Clinical presentation, Cardiovascular Pharmacotherapy International Symposium, Geneva, April 1985. Reported in Cardiology World News, Jan. 1986, p 29.
17. Small, patient-held monitor sends ECG results by phone. Cardiology World News July/Aug 1985, p 24.
18. Tzivoni D, Benhorin J, Gavish A, et al. Holter recording during treadmill testing in assessing myocardial ischemic changes. Am J Cardiol 55:1200–1203, 1985.
19. Lambert CR, Imperi GA, Pepine CJ. Low-frequency requirements for recording ischemic ST-segment abnormalities in coronary artery disease. Am J Cardiol 58:225–229, 1986.

Management

Chapter 11

Behavioral/Cognitive Interventions

Robert S. Eliot
Daniel Baker
Thomas Sawyer

Introduction

Most visits to physicians are not for actual physical complaints. Some are for information, some for reassurance, some for psychological concerns. In our culture, it is more acceptable to be physically sick than to have psychological distress, and therefore psychological distress is often masked as physical symptoms or illness. Therefore, like it or not, a physician often needs some skill in psychological assessment to determine the real reason for the patient's visit, the source of the distress, and the proper method of resolving the problem. With an understanding of basic behavioral approaches, health professionals can frequently help their patients deal with the stresses of ordinary life or the behavioral changes necessitated by physical illness.

Much of the information of a psychological nature can be obtained from a careful and detailed history and by observations made during the physical evaluation. Suggestions as to the appropriate behavioral approaches can then be made in the final evaluation. Of course, patients with the more serious psychological problems will require the services of a specialist, but those with problems less deeply ingrained, such as a

From: Eliot, RS: *Stress and the Heart: Mechanisms, Measurements and Management*. Mount Kisco, NY, Futura Publishing Company, Inc., © 1988.

post-MI patient without physical complications, probably will rely on their physicians for this type of guidance.

The following describes the methods used by the psychologists at our Center which can be adapted to various applications by the physician who works without a behavioral colleague.

Is Therapy Needed?

The first priority in the initial interview is to put the patient at ease. This can be done with humor, or completely mundane nonpejorative exchanges such as "What is the concern that brings you here today?" The next step is to draw out information relating to the three major areas: work, family, and personal life, including habits, behavior and beliefs across each of these three areas.

Often the patient will indicate in the course of the conversation what he is especially concerned about. This is then discussed in more depth, and the psychological assessment becomes somewhat of a counseling session. Once the scope of the problem is determined, the next question is how the patient is attempting to cope with it (sources of support, problem-solving style, coping style, resiliance, etc.). As was described, in our clinic, we have an integrated system in which psychologists perform this service.

While many people come to us because they feel that they are distressed, many don't know what stress is and are completely unaware of their stresses. If people are asked to rate their overall level of stress on a 0–5 scale, an answer of either 0 or 5 is cause for concern. If they say 5, it is evident that they need help with the stress load. If they say zero, either they don't know what stress is, or they are using strong denial systems. After all, we are all under commonly shared stresses of gravity, aging, traffic jams, deadlines of one sort or another, etc.

Critical factors are the degree of vigilance and control manifested in each of the three areas—work, family, and personal life.

With regard to vigilance: Are they constantly looking over a shoulder at how family members or subordinates are carrying out functions or at the boss to see if he or she approves, or at customers in fear of losing business?

With regard to control: How much control do they demand? Some act as if they should be the center of the universe. If they do not get the expected response, they feel that life is "unfair" and that they have lost control.

The primary issue in the personal area is one's health. Also, we look for stress management strategies; that is, how people react when they experience pressure. Obviously if their method of coping is to have a martini, it does not require a psychiatrist to see the warning sign. An increase in arguments and interpersonal conflicts is another important clue. Excessive sleep or disrupted sleep patterns are a meaningful sign. Indeed many physical symptoms suggest behavioral roots: asthma attacks, bronchitis, angina, gastrointestinal upset, headache, palpitations, tachycardia, abnormal eating patterns, light-headedness, dizziness, hyperventilation, shortness of breath, sense of unusual fatigue, etc. The patient's subjective feelings of anxiety, irritability, hostility, or depression clearly indicate distress. We especially look for unexpressed emotions of all types because these are often associated with metabolic and physiologic disruptions leading to ill health.

Because many of our patients are self-referred, they rarely disguise their perceived stress. Usually, it is so thinly veiled that it is easy to discern. Of course, if a person feels his problems will become known and possibly undermine his position at work, he may not be candid. Assurances of confidentiality are essential.

Stresses in the work area may involve relationships with peers, subordinates, superiors, or clients. Ask if any of these persons are particular standouts in accomplishment, or are personally abrasive. Does the patient feel comfortable in his position, or is he thwarted, misunderstood, or unappreciated? Does he have a briefcase in his head, i.e. tend to take the office everywhere with him (a sign of vigilance)?

Stresses in the family area may concern children, spouse, parents, in-laws, other close relationships, sexual problems, etc. Because sex is a particularly sensitive area, as well as a very important one, the physician should attempt to open up the subject in a tactful way. Chapter 15 describes various approaches in more detail.

With regard to children, are the children doing well? Are they having trouble finding their niche? Are there concerns with drugs? Are the children rebellious? Are they underachievers? Is there a mismatch between the parental expectations and the children's behavior?

Parents or other relatives may be sources of stress by being over-dependent or in poor health. Relationships with in-laws may be a problem.

In the personal area, the midlife crisis of males is a particularly common source of stress. This is revealed by a heightened consciousness of age. They are aware that they haven't achieved some of the goals that they had set for themselves. However, hobbies, interests, and friendships can be mitigating factors. These allow a person to disconnect from perpetual problem-solving. Without them it is easy to overload the internal computers that run day and night. A forty-year-old man with no hobbies or friends, no outlets, should be cause for concern. Having ways to let go is very important for managing stress.

Note whether the patient tends to blame others for problems. Blame is sometimes a symptom of deeper problems. Look for the "on-call" syndrome such as a startle whenever the phone rings (frequently observed in physicians). Look for hidden anger. Anger is often a secondary emotion; behind it is either hurt, frustration, anxiety, depression, or fear. If you are hurt, you may become angry to protect yourself; or if you are fearful, you are trying to confront the perceived threat.

Perfectionism is yet another indicator; achievement in this situation is not seen as a positive factor; it may occur because it is seen as the only alternative to failure. Perfectionism implies an *avoidance* factor, namely fear of failure. For instance, a person may rise to the presidency only to avoid remaining a vice-president, which would be perceived as failure or as having inadequate control. Avoidance is moving away from something—getting A's to avoid getting B's; not celebrating a win because you must concentrate on not losing the next one. Any failure would mean "I am a failure; hence, I am no good; I am a bad person . . ." Dwelling too much on a problem is an indication of distress; for instance, if a person wakes up ruminating on his work situation or other problem it is a sign of overload. One has to be able to disconnect from problems. We teach "active-detachment." That is, when progress can be made, work at it; when work becomes a struggle, detach, reflect, and reorganize, or await a more timely opportunity.

The written tests our patients are asked to take give us some insight into the sorts of difficulties the person may be experiencing.

The Quality of Life Index is a mixed bag of psychosocial variables that help greatly in giving patient, physician, and therapist insight into the perceived struggles and support systems of a person. It provides situations, behaviors, and character types with which people identify. For example, a person with time problems is like a Perpetual Pusher who says "hurry, hurry, hurry . . . gotta, gotta, gotta, . . . have to, have to, have to . . ." Like the white rabbit in Alice in Wonderland, "I'm late, I'm late . . ." A person with extreme circuit overload is one who says "I'll do it, I'll take the responsibility." Like a white knight, he'll do it because nobody else can. He feels everyone depends on him, and he must come through regardless of his own health, family relationships, etc. Supermom and Superdad fit here also.

The Multiple Affect Adjective Checklist (MAACL)[1] is another useful test because it gives indices for anxiety, depression, and hostility, three factors that are very important. It consists of 132 adjectives arranged alphabetically in three columns. The patients mark the words that describe how they generally feel. The words include positive feelings such as "agreeable," "tender," and "safe"; and negative ones such as "angry," "sad," and "terrible." Hostility is measured by 28 adjectives, anxiety by 21, and depression by 40. The rest are buffer items. Scoring is supposed to indicate a personality trait rather than a transient state. However, the test-retest reliability is reportedly about .68 for the anxiety scale after a seven-day interval.

The Eysenck Personality Inventory[2] consists of 57 questions to be answered Yes or No. It measures two personality dimensions: extroversion and neuroticism. It has been used mainly in research, and it is not validated as a diagonostic tool for psychiatric disorders. Nevertheless, it is a quick way to gain insights into a patient's general personality and may provide some clues to possible stressors. We define neuroticism as a the use of outmoded, traditional solutions for contemporary problems. Clearly this can lead to unnecessary struggle, anxiety, and perceived loss.

These tests, like all other subjective tests, are not 100% accurate, of course, as a person's scores may not entirely reflect his true state. However, impressions gained from such tests, the lifestyle questionnaire, and the personal interview, taken together, provide valuable psychological information to be weighed with the rest of the data on the patient.

Modes of Therapy

Our psychologists emphasize the cognitive aspects of behavior—thought processes, belief systems, and attitudes—but also blend in other approaches according to the needs of the individual patient. The patient and therapist first agree on what is to be accomplished, determine possible steps to reach the goal, and analyze any stumbling blocks that are perceived or encountered.

The therapy may be reevaluated and modified along the way as seems appropriate. Although the initial goals tend to be specific, such as reducing blood pressure or managing eating disorders, the therapist also endeavors to teach self-regulation in the broader context through problem-solving techniques and coping methods that have general applicability.

Rational Emotive Therapy

Rational emotive therapy (RET) emphasizes the cognitive aspects of life. It teaches people how to see the world more accurately in a less threatening way. To help people to identify their own distorted thinking we sometimes give them a pamphlet describing 15 styles of distorted thinking and ask them to put a check mark next to any categories that relate to their own cognitive practices.

The list includes the following[3]:

1. Filtering—a sort of tunnel vision, where one element of a situation is emphasized to the exclusion of everything else.

2. Polarized Thinking—the world is dichotomized into black and white, good and bad; extremes with no middle ground.

3. Overgeneralization or Hyperbolizing—one incident is distorted into generalized conclusion. Cue words are all, every, none, never, always, everybody, and nobody.

4. Mind Reading—assumptions are made as to what other people are feeling or thinking, based on what one would feel and think in the same situation.

5. Catastrophizing—assuming the worst possible outcome from a situation. Cue words "what if."

6. Personalization—the tendency to relate everything to oneself, measuring oneself against others, or interpreting every experience or conversation as a clue to one's own worth and value.

7. Control Fallacies—either seeing oneself as helpless and externally controlled, or as omnipotent and responsible for everyone else around.

8. Fallacy of Fairness—assuming that others should act fairly although fairness, being purely subjective, is rarely interpreted the same way by any two people.

9. Emotional Reasoning—thinking that all the negative self-evaluations must be true. ("If I feel ugly, then I must be ugly.")

10. Fallacy of Change—assuming that one's happiness depends on others changing in certain ways. Strategies used to change others include blaming, demanding, withholding, and trading.

11. Global Labeling—generalizing one or two qualities into a global judgment, resulting in a stereotyped, one-dimensional view of the world. (A person who refuses to provide a lift home is labeled a total jerk.)

12. Blaming—making someone else responsible for choices and decisions that are actually one's own responsibility; or conversely taking all the blame on oneself.

13. Shoulds—inflexible rules to determine the behavior of oneself and others. But judgments are not determined objectively and may make no sense.

14. Being Right—the need to always be right—defending a viewpoint but disregarding information that doesn't fit preconceived notions.

15. Heaven's Reward Fallacy—doing the "right thing" in hope of a reward or appreciation but becoming hostile when the reward does not come.

This list is not all-inclusive but contains those that are most common in our experience.

To see how such distorted thinking leads to stress, take, for example, the fallacy of fairness. No two people see things in the same way, so there can be no agreement as to what constitutes "fairness." Therefore, if one expects the world to be fair there will inevitably be disappointment.

There are three general sources of stress: the environment, (heat, pollen, dirt, etc.), the body (backaches, cold symptoms, etc.), and thoughts. Distorted thinking is probably the major source of stress, because it can create stress, and one's cognition is present at all times. All the events that occur are colored by a person's perception, and this is determined by the words or images in his/her mind.

For instance, when there is an accident or a relative dies, a person may react by thinking "This is awful, I can't stand it." But of course he can and is standing it. Or he thinks, "This shouldn't have happened." Yet all the prerequisites must have been present or it would not have happened; therefore, it had to—it "should"—happen. He may think, "I don't deserve this;" an example of the fallacy of fairness—that one's behavior should be rewarded appropriately by Heaven.

The "shoulds" indicate demandingness, a stress producer. According to the dictionary, "must" is an imperative requirement; a situation with no alternative. The word is frequently used inaccurately for situations that do have alternatives. "I must go to work." "I can't get out of this relationship." Such thoughts set up unnecessary inflexibility in a situation and create stress. The demandingness of "should," "must," "have to" leads to disappointment and invisible entrapment. Understanding this and learning to use more accurate language can alleviate a lot of stress.

"Should" is also misused as a future tense. "The bus should be here by now." Obviously, if traffic is heavy or there is mechanical difficulty, it "should" be late; all the prerequisites for lateness have been met.

People who look back at the past have the opportunity to learn from their mistakes, but some distort the past into a source of stress by the "if only" syndrome. "If only I hadn't worked so hard and spent more time with my son . . ." The "if only" is the past tense of the catastrophizing "what if." It is a tremendous waste of psychological energy to beat oneself over the head with things that cannot be changed. Instead, the energy could be better invested where changes are possible.

Such wastes of psychological energy can bankrupt one's supply and lead to the total personality collapse laymen call "a nervous break-down." Too often people assume that their emotional bank account is infinite just because they cannot assign numbers to the withdrawals. They then play fast and loose with their feelings.

But there cannot be feelings without thought, though it may appear so because of its brevity and rapidity. This is easily demonstrated by asking patients to "feel happy." They may find this difficult; but they easily follow the direction to "think of an event that made you feel particularly happy." Clearly feelings are determined by thoughts turned into neurophysiological prescriptions coming from the brain. Thoughts like "I am a loser," cause bad feelings. Thoughts like "I did well," generate good feelings. A positive way to handle a bad experience might be to reflect that "I paid a significant price for this experience—what have I learned?" instead of merely lamenting "This is horrible, this is terrible!"

Another problem is the confusion of approval with acceptance. A person may say "I cannot accept this situation," when he really means he disapproves of the situation. And if people understand the reality of the situation, that they must accept it and adjust to it, whether or not they approve, they narrow the gap between reality and their expectations. If they do not accept reality, the gap widens.

The brain can be likened to a sophisticated computer that everyone receives without an enclosed operator's manual. In a sense, cognitive therapy provides the manual on how to use it more accurately and effectively. We teach people to say what they mean and mean what they say. Otherwise, if they say what they don't mean, there is room for erroneous and irrational thinking, and the gap between reality and perception again widens. Distorted thinking leads to extreme reaction, beyond what is necessary or appropriate. Just as paying $2 for a tube of toothpaste marked $1 is overpayment, distorted thinking leads to overpayment physiologically, metabolically, and behaviorally.

Cognitive Restructuring

One exercise we give patients introduces them to a number of different belief systems that may be setting them up for problems. Awareness of the belief systems that underlie people's thinking can help them appreciate the origin of their negative feelings. The reason people are not conscious of their belief systems is that they have been so well practiced that they have become automatic. We try to bring these subconscious products of the limbic portion of the brain back to conscious levels. Habit, on the whole, is helpful; it permits the actions needed for common activities such as taking a key out of one's pocket to unlock a door or brushing the teeth to be performed reflexively without cumbersome step-by-step decisions. But some habits are harmful and just as automatic.

To illustrate this, patients are asked to name the color of the dictaphone. Immediately they respond "black." Then we point out that that is just how fast our cognitive apparatus responds to events in our lives. In the A,B,C's of an emotion, the A, activating event, falsely appears to cause C, the emotion that is the consequence of the event. But it is the B's (beliefs) that color perception and determine responses, and they are so rapid, so subtle, and so silent, that they appear to be absent. Automatic cognition, then, has to be brought up to the conscious level. *That requires concentrated thought and effort.* To illustrate the difficulty of changing such an ingrained habit, we may ask a patient to clasp his/her hands together in a different way from the habitual one, with the other hand in the superior position. See Figure 1.

In essence we ask patients to identify a few of the distorted B's that get them into trouble, that set them up for seeing saber-toothed tigers around every corner, or that cause self-blame. The A's have very little to do with the reaction except to dictate whether the event is positive or negative. A healthy internal tape would recognize and accept that life is a series of events, some positive, and some negative; then congruence with reality would be quite good. If it is understood that a few painful events are expected in normal life, then when one happens, it can be accepted, not misconstrued as a special punishment.

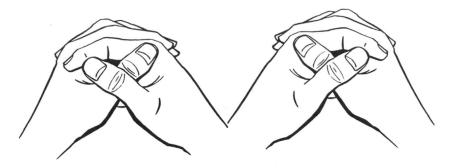

Figure 1: The way you fold your hands is an ingrained habit that is hard to change. At first it takes time and thought to fold them the opposite way, with the other thumb on top, but with practice it becomes easier. The same is true with changing self-talks and other habits.

On the other hand, we sometimes find a distorted pattern of "I am special; I shouldn't have any pain," or "I should be able to control things so I will be spared pain,"—an extreme form of omnipotency. While money, properly used, can be a coping resource, it is obvious from some wealthy patients we have seen that money is not always the key to controlling what happens to them. We teach people how to rearrange their internal world as opposed to trying to arrange the external world over which control is more limited. What good is lifestyle without life?

Some cognitive strategies work very quickly, unlike the Freudian type of analysis. If patients are motivated to examine their thinking patterns, they can continue the process of making their thoughts and statements more rational and effective on their own.

It takes only about three hours to teach the essence of the cognitive approach. It may take longer for the patient to develop new habits and resist falling back into old patterns. Any learning experience requires reinforcement within six weeks.

Various "exercises" can be helpful and revealing. For instance, we may ask a patient to note during a day whether he/she or others use the words "should," "must," and "have to" incorrectly. On another day, the search may be for another type of distorted thinking. We suggest that patients examine their own thinking for the types of beliefs that are implied and then restate the irrational ones in more rational form. Another exercise is to have the patient compare his/her reacting style in a situation that was handled very well with another where the patient paid too high an emotional price, analyzing the underlying belief systems.

In the beginning, patients may pick up on only one or two of the B's (perceptions), just the tip of the iceberg. For instance, thinking "I really screwed up at work today," may also imply "I am a loser; I may lose my job; what will happen to the family if I can't support them, etc." As we work with a person and ask questions to bring hidden thoughts to the surface, we may find as many as 15 or 20 B's inherent in one response. Then it is possible to determine the logical consequences, the various C's. If underneath "I am a loser" is "what happens when I don't make it," "what happens if I lose my job," "I won't be able to pay for things," it reveals feelings of fear, loss, and inadequacy.

We try to discern whether there is distorted thinking in thoughts about oneself, thoughts about others, and thoughts about the world. Most fall into the four styles of "Horriblization," "Demandingness," "I-can't-stand-it-itis," and the damning or negating of oneself.

Irrational superstitions or magical thinking sometimes influence behavior even when they are recognized as meaningless on the conscious level. (For example, childhood avoidance of stepping on a crack that "breaks your mother's back," persists in some adults.)

Improving Coping Behavior

Coping strategies are another key to stress management. Effective coping can have a positive effect on health. Ineffective coping, such as smoking, drinking, and avoidance, can cause health problems and interfere with more adaptive behaviors. Because no one strategy is effective in every situation, increasing patients' coping resources can make them more effective copers. Coping resources may include problem-solving skills, material resources, social support, information seeking, modes for action inhibition, and humor.

Often people know what they want to achieve but don't know how to do it. We try to identify the block, to find the belief that keeps them from doing what they want to do. If the therapist can find the block and get rid of it, then it is much easier for the patient to understand how to achieve his goal.

Sometimes people try too hard and put pressure on themselves. They are afraid of failing; they become vigilant and then get discouraged by repeated failures. We advise such people to back off and prioritize and pace themselves rather than to keep beating themselves up. For instance, an individual trying to lose weight may notice that his pants are tight. He says to himself "I'm getting fat; I should lose weight." The "should" sets up a judgmental process in which self-esteem is tied to whether he loses weight or not. The "should" makes him seem a good person or bad person by whether he succeeds. The person goes on a diet and then is constantly vigilant because if he goes off he is a "bad" person. The vigilance puts pressure on the individual and the pressure builds and builds over time. The person may crave something he particularly loves, such as chocolate ice cream, but is constantly reminding himself that he must stick to his diet. "I've got to . . . I've got to . . . I've got to . . ." But finally the vigilance and pressure build up so much that in a moment of weakness, perhaps after a particularly tiring day, he heads right for the "forbidden" treat and binges. In transactional analysis, this is considered the "rebellious child" who reacts to the "punishing parent" who has been causing the vigilance and guilt. This pattern often contributes to the scenario of patients who lose considerable weight in the first few weeks of a diet and then gain it all back, perhaps even additional weight, in the next few weeks. Most patients gain back all they have lost within a year.

For this reason, we try to steer away from prescribing a practice in which the patient has "got to" do this or that. We may be setting them up for failure if they hear it as a message from a strong parent, thereby activating the rebellious child. Instead, we emphasize the teaching of how a person processes information.

The first step of the educational process is to stick with the facts. In the previous example, the fact is just that "my pants are tight," not that "I should lose weight." The next step is "what can I do about it?" If the answer is to eat less, the patient may be helped by first noting what precipitates his desire to eat. Keeping a diary for a few days of where he is and what he is doing when he gets the desire to eat may disclose the triggers involved. Many people use eating as a substitute for problem-solving. "When I'm lonely I eat." But of course, eating doesn't solve loneliness. Instead, the patient needs help in how to be more sociable. Or if the eating is tied to problems with a spouse, marital counseling may be in order. Understanding the mind-behavior communication (how we process information) is the key to correcting the problem. Fortunately, this often does not require an extended period of time. The insight allows people to understand their motivation and thereby unblocks the motivation that can help them to succeed.

The idea is to raise to the awareness level the subconscious motivation and the internal self-talks that lead to self-defeating behavior. By determining the patient's styles of coping, basic beliefs, and modes of interaction and how they were developed, it is possible to point out the implicit values and strengths as well as the stressors and problems with others that may result.

This system, which encompasses a person's whole lifestyle, discloses how everything fits together—the behavior, the relationships, the career choices, even their child-rearing habits. The patients see that no one thing has an isolated effect, but that it all works together.

We aim for self-acceptance. It gets away from rating oneself, comparing oneself to others, making one's happiness dependent on measuring up to some elusive standard. We try to help each person to accept himself as a human being and not as a member of some profession or of a certain wealth.

Other Approaches

Because thoughts are always with us, cognitive restructuring is the most important method of reducing stress. Progressive muscle relaxation, biofeedback, and imagery have more limited utility. They mainly aid rest at night and help to rejuvenate one during breaks in the daytime routine.

Instead of conversation, acting out situations may be more meaningful to patients who are not particularly word oriented. Many male executives think in very concrete terms and so they are helped by being given very concrete examples of things to do. For instance, one manager who had to give a lot of presentations claimed he was basically shy and felt inadequate and tense when standing in front of a group of executives. The therapist suggested that he imagine them all sitting there in their underwear so they would appear less intimidating. He found this thought quite humorous and beneficial.

In stress management, such people respond better when they can see objective evidence of their relaxation, such as blood pressure dropping, etc. Thus, biofeedback may be a suitable adjunct with cognitive therapy. They require visual evidence of physical changes because they are not very well in touch with their own bodies, tending to deny the discomforts or tenseness that others are aware of.

On the other hand, with a person who is more imaginative and thinks more abstractly, we discuss values and beliefs, the part these play in creating stress, and how the conflicts can be resolved. We can use relaxation techniques without special equipment for these people because they are able to determine how they are doing by their own sensations.

Animal experiments have shown that stress associated with novel situations often decreases after several repetitions. This is true of humans as well and explains why blood pressure readings may be markedly higher when first taken than on the third or fourth try during an office visit. Patients anticipating surgery may feel less apprehensive if they are given some idea (but not all the gory details) of what to expect: the presurgical measures, the hospital routine, the purposes and effects of medications and tests, the expected discomforts and what can be done about them, etc.

Rehearsals of difficult times in daily life also can help to relieve some of the stress. For instance, a man who has stopped smoking might anticipate the situations when he will be most tempted to smoke and figure out how best to handle them. What will he say if a colleague offers him a cigarette while they are chatting over coffee? How will he control his nervousness while sitting waiting for an important interview? Imagining such scenes is useful, but actually acting them out in a controlled situation with a counselor or supportive friend may be necessary to convince some patients that they can really remain in control.

Such rehearsals can help to maintain compliance. Some patients need a very structured relapse-prevention program. For instance, hospital patients who have been having daily sessions for about two weeks, may need guidance before discharge in how to handle situations at home. It is important for a counselor to discuss the situations and difficulties that are likely to give them problems. "What are you going to do when that happens?" The patients are reminded of what they have been taught, and they visualize themselves coping in the new way.

We do the same sort of thing with hypertensive patients. We often tell them at the last session, "This is something you need to understand: it is highly likely that some time in the next six months that you will have the tendency to start relapsing. It is not a time to panic. Go back to what brought you here and remember what you did to enable you to successfully control your blood pressure. You are guarding against vigilant behaviors, pacing yourself at work, and practicing your relaxation skills. If your blood pressure starts to go up you are undoubtedly neglecting one or all three of those things. So you don't even need to call us. You already know what to do. However, if you get back on the program and your blood pressure is still up, then call."

We don't want people to become dependent and to feel that a physician or psychologist is needed to get them through every difficulty. Instead we try to teach them how to solve problems themselves. It is analagous to giving a hungry person a fishing pole instead of a fish. They must learn how to make it on their own.

Awareness is the first step in therapy. With further counseling sessions, it is possible to focus on specific problems and zero in on strategies that can be implemented to resolve those problems. For instance, some hypertensive executives may be uptight in dealing with authority figures. They feel they are undeserving of their position; underneath they feel shy and unworthy. This is stressful. They may then be too deferential to their supervisors, perhaps working overtime to the detriment of their marriage or health. Then we help them work on becoming more assertive, putting reasonable and prudent limits on the control by the boss.

Blood Pressure Management

People have their highest blood pressure when they are most vigilant. A salesman will be most vigilant when he is talking to clients on the telephone and have highest pressure at such times. A computer programmer will have his highest pressure while studying the computer screen intently. If someone is driving on the freeway and is watching anxiously for other drivers trying to get ahead of him, that is when his pressure will be highest.

Identifying the times of greatest vigilance is the key to controlling the highest blood pressures. The simple action of breathing properly at such times can help lower the blood pressure and reduce the risk.

We use a three-pronged approach for behavioral control of blood pressure: (1) building awareness of the stress triggers; (2) teaching strategies for interrupting the stress cycle; (3) modifying behavior that accentuates the stress reaction.

An important part of the therapy is to teach the patient proper breathing by means of biofeedback or relaxation or a combination of the two techniques. A second component is some strategy for interrupting the stress cycle. One strategy is the blue-dot system in which blue dots are pasted where they can be seen during times of stress. Rubber bands or other materials could also be used. The purpose is to use some stimulus or cue to remind the person to practice proper breathing. The blue-dot system is versatile because the dots can be placed on so many different things—rearview mirror of the car, watchface, telephone, etc. So every time the individual looks at his watch, he's reminded to take deep breaths. The object is to interrupt this stress cycle where everything goes faster, faster, faster. The more times that that cycle is disrupted, the slower and less tense things tend to be.

We have our patients look at the pace and rhythms of their walking, talking, and eating behaviors. For instance, many people who are hypertensive tend to walk fast, talk fast, and eat fast. So, we'll try to modify these behaviors. The treatment plan incorporates all these goals: biofeedback to help them to reduce their vigilance and reactiveness to situations; some behavior modification, substituting behaviors that don't perpetuate that stress cycle; and enhanced awareness of unnecessary vigilance—the behaviors that get them into the most trouble—with supportive reminding to break up the stress cycle. Remember, simplistic Johnny-One-Note approaches usually fail, whereas orchestrations have a good chance of success.

Compliance

Compliance is one of the top problems in behavioral therapy today. There is a tendency for relapse. It depends a lot on individual makeup and motivation. With SHAPE patients, much of the material on cognitive restructuring is covered in the final discussion. This conversation is taped and the cassette is given to the patient. Patients are requested to play the tape of "The Final" the next day after their analysis, then a week later, the next month, in three months, and again six months later. We also suggest that the "significant other" listen to it too. This replay really provides reinforcement for change. However, without follow-up it is difficult to motivate some patients to continue with the therapy. A workbook[4] and frequent reinforcing phone calls have been successful in aiding compliance. The phone calls may be no longer than ten or fifteen minutes, just to check on progress, answer a few questions, and offer continuing encouragement.

Often when the physician points out how stress is leading to serious or manifest physical problems such as hypertension, ulcers, or decreased immune function, the patient will be amenable to seeing a psychologist or psychiatrist for "stress management," although he/she would not consider going for "counseling" or "psychotherapy."

A patient who wants to learn a nonpharmacologic way to manage blood pressure must be willing to come to at least four sessions. Compliance is a function of how well the expectations of the patient and the expectations of the therapist match. After four sessions, the therapist can evaluate the progress. If what has been accomplished is helpful but is not finished, the patient may be asked to commit to four more sessions. If these are not helpful, the patient and therapist will shake hands and part company amicably. If it is foreseen that a serious longer term problem exists, the therapist can explain this and inform the patient that he needs someone he can better relate to for the longer-term therapy or for pharmacologic management. With the "well walking wounded" we can do a lot in four to eight sessions.

The role of the therapist is that of a teacher who can suggest certain things to patients. If the patients don't cooperate, however, they are only wasting our time and their money. Patients have to take the ultimate responsibility for their own blood pressure and decide whether it is a priority for them. The therapist may dangle the carrot and say "If you make your health a priority for the next eight weeks, I think you will feel good enough and so encouraged by what you are accomplishing that you will want to continue it." However, it is important to learn the patient's motivation. If he says, "I'm here because my doctor told me to come," or "because my wife said she would leave me otherwise," that is quite different from a motivation stemming from the belief that he can be helped. We don't create the sham that they are getting better just because they are seeing a psychologist when all they are doing is trying to appease somebody else. This is just lateralling the ball behind the line of scrimmage.

The proof of their compliant attitude is not what they say but what they do. The relaxation techniques require practice twice a day to develop the skill, and it is usually easy to tell by the level of improvement whether a patient has been practicing faithfully or not. If they do not comply, we suggest they discuss alternative treatments or medications with their physician. After about three or four sessions, if the therapist has not enlisted the patient's cooperation and built a rapport, it is not going to happen in six or eight.

After patients have had some success, they may return less frequently. Usually if they continue to do well after several evaluative sessions, they go on an "as needed" basis. They are told to call when they feel they need to talk to or visit the therapist. Basically, however, they are informed that they don't need a regularly scheduled therapy session. Then when they do call, the psychologist judges whether a visit is necessary. It is similar to dancing with a partner: you have to sense when it is time to lead, when to follow. You move as they are moving. If they are moving well, you get out of the way. If they are not moving well you will be more directive and active.

Efficacy

No therapy has a great track record for weight reduction. Of the therapies that have been tried, cognitive therapy may be the best. In our experience, for depression cognitive therapy has a much better track record and, together with chemotherapy when it is needed, is the best treatment for this condition.

Cognitive therapy, as with other therapies, is more effective with the higher socioeconomic levels than with the lower ones and works best with those more comfortable with abstractions. Because some people require a more concrete approach, therapy that is very structured and direct works best with them. On the other end of the scale are people who can deal with the abstract; they philosophize, and the therapist can be much more insight-oriented with them. The cognitive behavioral therapy is not one-dimensional; it can blend or flow toward the behavioral. With the lower socioeconomic groups we tend to be more behavioral and less cognitive. With those from upper socioeconomic groups we tend to be more cognitive and less behavioral.

Cognitive approaches are less successful with the elderly, the less verbal, lower intellectual groups, but they are less apt to seek help anyway. For them it may be more effective to use social and economic policy to influence behavior. For instance, they are more likely to be helped if approached through their place of employment than on a one-to-one basis.

In my view, if it were socially acceptable for persons to back away from responsibility occasionally and take a break and rest for legitimate psychological reasons instead of for physical reasons only, there would be less illness. This is well illustrated in the phenomenon of posttraumatic stress disorder. Persons who have a frightening experience without physical injury may have longer-lasting mental trauma than those who have the same experience with physical injury that permits them to get extra rest, sympathetic attention, and acceptable regression into invalidism. Too often, these victims may be shunted from physician to physician only to be told there is nothing wrong with them, instead of being helped. It may only be years later, when the situation is in litigation, that a psychiatrist will be called in for the purpose of preparing a court case.[5]

It has been our experience that psychologists trained in behavioral medicine, usually require only a few weeks to obtain meaningful results with stressed patients. Long expensive therapy extending over more than three months is the exception. *The key to success is practice,* with many repetitions of the desired mode of thinking or behaving in order to establish new habits. Behavioral therapy can be as potent as pharmacological therapy, and a behavioral psychologist or psychiatrist working on the team with a patient's personal physician provides optimal benefit.

References

1. Zuckerman M, Lubin B. Manual for the Multiple Affect Adjective Check List. Educational and Industrial Testing Service. San Diego, 1965.
2. Eysenck HJ, Eysenck SBJ. Manual. Eysenck Personality Inventory. Educational and Industrial Testing Service. San Diego, 1968.
3. McKay M. Thoughts and Feelings: The Art of Cognitive Stress Intervention. New Harbinger Publications, Richmond, CA, 1981.
4. Eliot RS, Breo DL. Is It Worth Dying For? Bantam Books, New York, 1984.
5. Modlin HC. Posttraumatic stress disorder: No longer just for war veterans. Postgrad Med 79(3):26–44, 1986.

Chapter 12

Pharmacological Treatment of Stress

Robert S. Eliot
Elizabeth Yaeger

Anxiety

Minor Tranquilizers—Benzodiazepines

For treating just anxiety without depression, all the minor tranquilizers are about equally effective. The choice will depend on the half-life desired. Diazepam (Valium) has a long half-life, and there is danger of buildup. Many also complain of side effects lingering beyond the anxiolytic effect. Alprazolam (Xanax), lorazepam (Ativan) and oxazepam (Serax) have short half-lives and are preferred for the elderly who are very susceptible to toxic buildup leading to the oversedated patient. On the other hand, if treatment with a short half-life is stopped too suddenly, the patient may experience seizures.[1] This can be avoided with proper tapering. If the patient cannot be trusted to take the medication as ordered it is best to use one with a long half-life as it will have a built-in tapering effect.

In the hospital, the short-acting ones would be preferred in most cases; but for home use, the patient's compliance behavior would determine which is preferable. We generally favor giving every MI patient a tranquilizer to prevent or relieve anxiety. Anxiety is such a provoker of

From: Eliot, RS: Stress and the Heart: Mechanisms, Measurements and Management. Mount Kisco, NY, Futura Publishing Company, Inc., © 1988.

epinephrine and norepinephrine both of which increase myocardial oxygen demands as delineated earlier. Excess catechols can lead to both contraction-band lesions (described earlier), infarct extension, and more infarcts. Alprazolam, our preferred choice, actually has been shown to decrease epinephrine and norepinephrine,[2] and it will not exacerbate an underlying depression as the other tranquilizers may do. It has a short half-life which also makes it suitable for out-patient management.

Alprazolam has some antidepressant side effects to it as compared to the other minor tranquilizers.[3] A person with a serious cardiovascular problem, whether it be arrhythmias, post by-pass, infarction, angina, silent ischemia, etc., can safely be treated with alprazolam which apparently has no cardiovascular side effects or interactions at all.[2] The usual antidepressant drugs have cardiovascular side effects and cannot be used for such patients.

Treatment post MI or by-pass may only be required for a few weeks. Ordinarily, if the anxiety and depression that follow by-pass or MI have not been resolved by 3 to 6 months, professional psychiatric care is indicated.

Side Effects

Occasionally, a patient shows a paradoxical reaction to a tranquilizer and becomes aroused and excited instead of being calmed.[4] The incidence is reported at 1% to 5%. If this happens, it is safe to change to another of the benzodiazepines unless there is an underlying depression. Sometimes several trials will be needed to find one that has the desired effect. A few people may show paradoxical reactions to all tranquilizers. It is best to utilize rather low doses for this trial period until one is seen to have a calming action.

There is always the possibility of addiction but this is not very likely unless the dosage has to be increased steadily. It is important to keep good records of dates and amounts of prescriptions for each individual for this reason. Most patients can be tapered off within days or a few weeks of some cardiovascular event. When those requiring longer management become stabilized, they can be gradually tapered off tranquilizers after six months. If they then become more anxious and have increased problems, we consider whether they are developing an agitated depression (and then treat that if present) or give them cognitive therapy pertinent to their current problems. We prefer this to increasing the dosage of a tranquilizer. We also require that the patient return every few months if refills are requested; phoned refills are well known to lead to dangerous situations. We warn the patients of the dangers of addiction and assure them that it is very unlikely if they follow instructions carefully.

The minor tranquilizers do not affect blood pressure, cause cardiovascular problems, or interact with the medications commonly prescribed for hypertension or diabetes. However, except for alprazolam, these drugs may increase the liver enzymes and increase the breakdown of other medications. It is important to be aware of this phenomenon since higher dosages may be required as is the case with warfarin (Coumadin).

Barbiturates

These agents are rarely used today because the minor tranquilizers are so much safer. In our view, the only indication for their use is for seizures or for people, less than six weeks post MI, who have rapid eye movement (REM) onset nightmares related to arrhythmias.[1,5] The barbiturates stop REM sleep and suppress dreaming. This gives the heart time to heal. Protracted suppression of REM sleep can, however, lead to a variety of psychotic states in susceptible individuals.

Depression

Depression is not uncommon following a cardiac event. However, depression can also result as a side effect of certain medications, and this possibility should be considered especially with patients receiving cimetidine, methyldopa, clonidine, guanethidine, or reserpine.[6]

Alprazolam (Xanax)

It is not safe to employ the usual antidepressant agents for at least six weeks after a by-pass or MI or for a patient having arrhythmias because of their adverse cardiac effects. Actually, these people do not generally go into a severe endogenous depression in the first six weeks —the sort where they lose their serotonin and norepinephrine, the neurotransmitters that help maintain normal mood. Usually we recommend using alprazolam. It is now being reviewed by the FDA for approval as an antidepressant, but it is already approved for anxiety (and such patients usually display a lot of anxiety). In trials it seems to be as effective as imipramine and produces its effect faster.[3]

Electroconvulsive Shock Treatment (ECT)

Besides alprazolam, the only other treatment for a significantly depressed patient with severe cardiovascular disease is electroconvulsive shock treatment (ECT). Some physicians believe this is actually the safest antidepressant for cardiovascular patients,[7] but the risk of anesthesia must be considered.

Tricyclic Antidepressants

For the majority of patients who do well on an exercise ECG, these agents are very useful in counteracting depression. They also decrease anxiety; so for someone with both anxiety and depression, they are helpful. However, they are not recommended within six weeks of MI or by-pass or for those with certain other cardiac problems because of the possibility of undesirable side effects.[8] As mentioned above, alprazolam can be used in this situation, and it does help. It is a matter of monitoring the patient and being aware of the risks. The physician must be very familiar with the state of the person's cardiovascular system as well as the person's psychological makeup. There is little value in a perfect cardiac rhythm if the patient takes a shotgun to his head.

ECG monitoring is important for any patient on tricyclics because of potential rhythm changes such as increased PR interval, widened QRS, or ST-T wave changes. Mainly the antidepressants seem to prolong the pre-ejection time and shorten the left ventricular ejection time. This has the overall effect of decreasing myocardial contractility and decreasing the pump action.

Certain tricyclics, such as amitriptyline and imipramine, can cause such problems as postural hypotension; this can decrease cardiac output thus worsening congestive heart failure. Recently thallium scan studies have revealed that this may be a concern for some people, although it may not cause problems for most. Nortriptyline is somewhat less apt to cause orthostatic hypotension than imiprimine.[9]

Some of the newer tricyclic antidepressants (amoxapine, trimipramine, maprotiline) have less effect on the cholinergic receptors and are less likely to induce arrhythmias that can lead to ventricular fibrillation. Sometimes a quinidinelike effect of tricyclics leads to decreased incidence and severity of arrhythmias. The problem is that a stabilized patient who stops taking the medication for some reason is subject to a rebound effect. Patients are urged to call us first if they wish to stop the medication in order that, at the very least, it can then be stopped gradually and with the least risk.

Tricyclics basically decrease blood pressure through direct peripheral vasodilation, secondary to decreasing cardiac output, which, in turn, is secondary to a decrease in cardiac contractility.

The hypotensive effect can be minimized by using divided doses instead of the one-a-day form. Doxepin has sometimes been characterized as less hypotensive,[7] but dosages that provide an antidepressant effect comparable to the other tricyclics also lead to the same problems. (Note: In our experience, 275 mg of Sinequan [doxepin] is probably equivalent to 200 mg of Elavil [amitriptyline]; not 200 mg = 200 mg as is sometimes stated.)

Among the antidepressants, the one with the least effect on the blood pressure is nortriptyline. The tetracyclic maprotiline is also less hypotensive. However, when dosage reaches about 225 mg, it frequently causes seizures.

Sometimes to help with the hypotension caused by the tricyclics, a little bit of thyroxine (Synthroid) could be added. In low doses (e.g., .05 mg) it will not necessarily cause increased heart rate, and it permits the use of less antidepressant. The receptors in the brain for serotonin and for norepinephrine, the primary antidepressant molecules, need to be readied by thyroxine. So giving them a little more has a potentiating effect.

The tricyclics, besides lowering blood pressure, which can cause an ischemic effect, also increase heart rate, which of course increases myocardial oxygen demand and can also cause ischemia. The increase is about 9 to 16 beats per minute, depending on the drug used. After the person has been stabilized on one of them (4 to 6 weeks), the heart rate usually returns to normal limits.[11]

The tertiary amines, like imipramine, affect the inward sodium current of the Purkinje fibers.[11] Lithium also has this effect. Caution is the byword, therefore, with manic/depressives who have cardiovascular disorders and who are taking either of these agents, in view of their effect on myocardial sodium and potassium concentrations.

It is necessary to ensure that the person does not have bundle branch block. Usually it is best to avoid antidepressants in the presence of bundle branch block. This may not be so true with some of the newer ones. The danger is that the block may go on to become a second or even third-degree heart block.[9,11]

Imipramine has a quinidinelike effect—it suppresses the ectopic pacemakers. When given to patients with pacemakers below the SA node, a tricyclic such as imipramine, may cause an idioventricular rhythm, and the person may even go into asystole. That is why it is essential to know where the blocks are. People who are receiving type I antiarrhythmic drugs like procainamide (Pronestyl) and quinidine should not be given tricyclics. But patients who are showing PVCs with a normal functioning SA node, often improve on the tricyclics.

Tricyclics, such as imipramine, can slow conduction through the heart and can even cause a dangerously high ventricular rate. For patients having this reaction, digitalis may be prescribed and then the tricyclics can be added.

Patients who have depressive states but are decompensating, with edema and congestive heart failure, should not be given the tricyclic antidepressants because they will probably get worse. It would be necessary to restrict their fluids, predisposing them to severe hypotension.

The tricyclics block the neural reuptake mechanism of norepinephrine and the action of acetylcholine.[1] As a result they can cause neural disturbances.

Some tricyclics may interact with other medications. For instance, when imipramine is used together with cimetidine (Tagamet), the cimetidine potentiates the imipramine and dosage must be carefully monitored to avoid toxicity. Doxepin and trimipramine decrease gastric acid secretion and block histamine. So for the depressed person with stomach problems, these can be used alone without the necessity for cimetidine. Doxepin also is effective in treating anxiety.

In summary, tricyclics should not be used:

1. Within 6 weeks of an infarction
2. In presence of congestive heart failure
3. In presence of decompensation
4. In presence of rhythm disturbances

They should be introduced slowly, and ECG's should be performed frequently, especially before each increase in dosage. The frequency of ECGs should depend on the perceived patient risk. For those who look good on treadmill ECG, and are well stabilized on drugs, every three or four months may be sufficient.

Trazodone

Trazodone (Desyrel) acts by inhibiting serotonin uptake. It has some hypotensive effect, but has almost no anticholinergic problems. It is contraindicated in persons with ventricular arrhythmias, as it can worsen this condition. Desipramine is better for such patients. Trazodone could be used on patients with PVCs if they don't have problematic arrhythmias. Trazodone is safe for the elderly, but some experience considerable sedation with it.[12]

Monoamine Oxidase Inhibitors

If a very depressed patient cannot use tricyclics because of cardiac problems and will not allow an ECT, one can employ a monoamine oxidase (MAO) inhibitor. This is possible only if the patient is cooperative and will maintain the necessary restrictions. As their name implies, these agents interfere with the enzyme that degrades serotonin and norepinephrine. However, to avoid precipitating a hypotensive crisis, patients must avoid foods containing tyramine (cheese, wine, pickled herring, etc.) as well as all decongestants. In other respects this is a very safe drug.

If hypotension becomes a problem, be certain the patient drinks plenty of fluid, maintains his/her weight, and uses some salt. We sometimes supplement with thyroid extract, a low dose of fludrocortisone acetate (Florinef), and a cup or two of regular coffee (not decaffeinated) as needed to stabilize the blood pressure.

Estrogen

In postmenopausal women, estrogen is very useful for counteracting depression. It can make a surprisingly big difference, such that no other antidepressant is required. Beware of the slightly increased risk of complications, such as thromboembolism and hypertension, this confers. The enhanced quality of life is worth the small gamble to most patients as the lowered cardiovascular risk may assist in counterbalancing the other factors.

The Elderly

The elderly have the most cardiovascular disease but have the most difficulty with medications. When the forward blood flow slows down, the kidneys, which have already lost nephrons, are not as well perfused, and renal insufficiencies progress further. Thus, the elderly are in danger of toxic buildup, and with tricyclics this can lead to arrhythmias, ventricular fibrillation and sudden death. Hypotension also predisposes them to falling, which causes bone fractures more often than would occur in younger patients. The break, in turn, can lead to a pulmonary embolism that may cause death. Even worse, head injury in an elderly patient often results in a subdural hematoma. (This danger is increased because, as the brain shrinks with age, a larger space is created between the brain and the skull.) Since it is likely that cerebrovascular disease is present along with cardiovascular disease, any significant uncompensated drop in blood pressure produces the possibility of stroke as well as of myocardial ischemia or infarction.

Ergoloid mesylates (hydergine), which is mainly used for improving memory in patients with Alzheimer's disease, has been found helpful also for depression in the elderly. It has fewer side effects than aspirin and is considered quite safe (although expensive). Its worst problem is possible gastrointestinal discomfort—diarrhea and nausea.[13]

Hypertensives

Many antihypertensive agents can cause depression. Methyldopa and reserpine are two antihypertensive medications that induce a lot of depression.[14] With clonidine, guanethidine, and propranolol, the incidence is about 1%, provided doses are moderate.

What about the patient who becomes depressed from taking an antihypertensive and, who, for various reasons, cannot take the alternative antihypertensives? In this case, an antidepressant can be added, but the patient must be cooperative, educated in the problems and limitations, and carefully monitored. Some depressed patients respond to large doses of tryptophane. This amino acid will not interfere with the anithypertensive medication and will help patients to sleep (a frequent application). If some of the other antidepressant drugs (especially tricyclics) are used with guanethidine and clonidine, the antihypertensives probably will not work as well.[15] There seems to be no problem in using antidepressants with diuretics, except for hypotension from volume depletion. Lanoxin and tricyclics are compatible.

If there is depression that precludes the use of tricyclics, it is possible to treat both the depression and the hypertension with MAO inhibitors, as long as the patient is careful to stay away from the tyramine foods, particularly cheese, beer, and wine. The MAO inhibitors are especially useful in persons with atypical depression—those with eating disorders, overeaters, the unmotivated, etc.[1]

Duration

It takes from four to six weeks for the antidepressants to take full effect and treatment generally continues for 6 to 12 months. Dosage is then gradually decreased over a period of about 4 weeks. But we do not start to taper them if we know there are high stress periods imminent (such as a wedding, a major work project, etc.). About a week after each decrease in dosage, one can observe whether the depression is returning. If so, resuming their original dosage usually produces a therapeutic effect within a few days, rather than the four to six weeks required in the initial treatment.

Psychosis

Major Tranquilizers

Major tranquilizers, the neuroleptics, are not often employed, mainly because of the risk of tardive dyskinesia. They are also apt to cause disturbances in ventricular repolarization with large doses, and it is suspected that ventricular arrhythmias related to their use may be the cause of the occasional sudden death during long-term treatment.[16]

If the patient does develop a psychosis, a low dosage of haloperidol (Haldol) may be prescribed. For ICU psychosis, 2 to 5 Haldol, three or four times a day, is generally sufficient. Haldol is the least detrimental to the cardiovascular system, but it does cause extrapyramidal effects, such as stiffness, nervousness, anxiety, restlessness, etc. and it may be necessary to use diphenhydramine (Benadryl) or benztropine mesylate (Cogentin) in addition.[1,3] Fortunately, the ICU problems generally clear up in a few days.

General Considerations

Because of the decreased activity of liver and kidney function in the elderly, all medications should be started at the minimal level and increased gradually. Precautions against overdosage should be taken. Once-a-day pills may be desirable to simplify the regimen. Pillboxes with the day and time indicated can be helpful. Overdosage of the minor tranquilizers can cause drowsiness; overdosage of the antidepressants can cause more serious effects. It may be preferable to have a companion or relative supervise the medications for an elderly person who has mental confusion.

It should be stressed to all patients not to discontinue their medications suddenly, but instead to taper off. They should be informed of the various alternative names for the same drug, because some pharmacies make substitutions, and patients may worry that they have received the wrong thing.

Patients should also be forewarned of common side effects and given suggestions for management. In addition, they should be told what signs to report immediately.

In depression and other severe mental conditions, it is my policy to ask for a psychiatric opinion before referring the patient for psychologic therapy. The risk of suicide or potential violence from psychotic breaks and the frequent need for medications preclude initial nonpharmacologic (psychologic) management in my view.

References

1. Gold M, Lydiard RB, Carman J. Advances in Psychopharmacology: Predicting and Improving Treatment Response. CRC Press, Boca Ratan, Fla, 1984.
2. Stratton JR, Halter JB. Effect of a benzodiazepine (alprazolam) on plasma epinephrine and norepinephrine levels during exercise stress. Am J Cardiol 56:136–139, 1985.
3. Feighner JP, Aden GC, Fabre LF, et al. Comparison of alprazolam, imipramine, and placebo in the treatment of depression. JAMA 249:3057–3064, 1983.
4. Weber RJ, Oszko MA, Bolender BJ, et al. The intensive care unit syndrome: causes, treatment, and prevention. Drug Intell Clin Phar 19:13–20, 1985.
5. Karacan I, Eliot RS, Dace M, et al. Nocturnal angina pectoris in relation to sleep and dreaming. The J Fla Med Assoc 55:348, 1968.

6. Ouslander JG, Small GW. Management of depression in the elderly patient with physical illness. Geriatric Med Today 3(10):90–96, 1984.
7. Neshkes RE, Jarvik LF. Depression in the elderly: current management concepts. Geriatrics 41(9):51–58, 1986.
8. Hollister LE. Psychiatric disorders. In: Avery GS (ed). Drug Treatment: Principles and Practice of Clinical Pharmacology and Therapeutiocs. Adis Press, New York, 1980.
9. Roose SP, Glassman AH, Giardina EGV, et al. Tricyclic antidepressants in depressed patients with cardiac conduction disease. Arch Gen Psychiatry 44:273–275, 1987.
10. Luchins DJ. Review of clinical and animal studies comparing the cardiovascular effects of doxepin and other tricyclic antidepressants. Am J Psychiatry 140(8):1006–1009, 1983.
11. Glassman AH, Bigger JT Jr. Cardiovascular effects of therapeutic doses of tricyclic depressants. Arch Gen Psych 38:815–820, 1981.
12. Lazarus LW, Davis JM, Dysken MW. Geriatric depression: A guide to successful therapy. Geriatrics 40(6):43–53, 1985.
13. McEvoy GK (ed). Drug Information 85. American Society of Hospital Pharmacists, Bethesda, Md. 1985. pp 509–510.
14. Haber E, Slater EE. High blood pressure. Section 1.VII in Sci Am Med. 4/86.
15. Rush DR. Drug interactions: when patients take antihypertensives. Diagnosis 8(4):113–123, 1986.
16. AMA Drug Evaluations, 5th ed.

Chapter 13

Antihypertensive Medications

Robert S. Eliot
Hugo Morales-Ballejo

Hypertension is now recognized as being enormously heteroge-
neous, both clinically and prognostically. Treatment must be correlated
with diverse factors. Our hemodynamic approach to treatment considers first of all whether cardiac output, total systemic resistance or
both need to be reduced. Medication of the appropriate type diminishes
side effects and enhances compliance. In our experience, using this
system, only about one treated and "controlled" patient in seven is
really hemodynamically controlled; six of seven are only "cosmetically"
controlled. The choice of therapeutic agent within each hemodynamic
category also must be individualized.

No medication is without possible side effects and, since the treatment of hypertension tends to be a long-term commitment, we strongly
advocate nonpharmacological treatment wherever possible, and no
treatment where benefit does not outweigh risks or adverse effects.
Afterall, reduction of elevated blood pressure does not prevent stroke or
coronary heart disease to the same degree that an immunization prevents an infectious disease. Treatment may be effective in preventing a
large *number* of adverse events, such as strokes; nevertheless, as many
or more such events will occur in treated patients and there is no clear
indication as to which individual hypertensive will benefit. Antihypertensive management to date has made only a minor dent in coronary
heart disease or sudden cardiac death.

From: Eliot, RS: *Stress and the Heart: Mechanisms, Measurements and Management.* Mount
Kisco, NY, Futura Publishing Company, Inc., © 1988.

The impact of medication on quality of life and the likelihood of patient compliance must be considered as well as the probability of benefit. The physician must be aware of how the patient's age, family history, risk factors, or coexisting conditions impact on therapeutic goals and methods. Alcohol use should also be noted, as excessive alcohol intake raises the blood pressure.

For instance, a young asymptomatic male with mild hypertension would be treated as a precaution to prevent later morbidity and mortality from cardiovascular causes. If he smokes, beta blockers may not provide any protection from strokes or coronary events.[1] A diuretic may be somewhat more effective, but if he experiences impotency, he may stop taking it. A fragile elderly woman given a drug, such as prazosin, that tends to cause hypotension and dizziness may be more at risk from sustaining head injuries or hip fractures due to falls than from the sequelae of hypertension.

Since hypertension involves long-term therapy, compliance is a major consideration in achieving control. Obviously cost is not a minor consideration in many cases. Although the physician may prefer one of the newer drugs because of milder or less frequent side effects, it may be worthwhile to try a less expensive alternative, if the cost is a limiting factor for the individual. The patient could be warned of the tradeoff and assured that another medication could be tried if side effects of the first one prove to be unacceptable.

Monotherapy, custom-tailored to the hemodynamic abnormalities, can be given at doses below the level that causes side effects, and the simplest treatment schedule are desirable. Combination of low doses of two drugs to obviate side effects, however, is often the best option. It has been noted that patients receiving more than three medications frequently make errors in taking them.[2] Interactions between drugs are also more likely the more complex the overall treatment becomes.

Who Should Not Receive Medication

Most Mild Hypertensives

The Medical Research Council trial[1] revealed that over time, blood pressure decreased in many of the placebo group of mild hypertensives. Cardiovascular events tended to cluster in the 12% whose blood pressures rose during the first three months of the trial. Blood pressure can be affected by temporary stresses, even the unfamiliarity with the procedure (white coat syndrome). Therefore, unless the hypertension is severe, it is advisable to monitor patients periodically for three or four months before instituting pharmacologic therapy.[3] Fortunately, in many instances blood pressure will drop without treatment or with nonpharmacological therapy.

Nonsmoking Premenopausal Women

For premenopausal women, the risk of cardiovascular events is very low even at severe levels of blood pressure except for diabetics and for smokers on birth control pills. Even the latter would be better off giving up smoking (or pills) rather than starting on a regimen of antihypertensive medication. Diabetics too, with mild hypertension, should try to lose weight and cut down on salt before instituting drug therapy that may add to their metabolic control problems. In one study[4] treatment of hypertensive women (SBP > 159, or DBP > 94) did not reduce the six-year incidence of CHD below that expected in relation to the pretreatment blood pressure.

When Quality of Life Suffers

In reviewing the benefits of lowering blood pressure, Dollery[5] noted that controlling blood pressure did not seem to completely reverse the adverse prognosis. The drug used to control the pressure, as well as the degree of control, was noted to affect the subsequent incidence of strokes or myocardial infarction. Stroke prevention was more effective with diuretics than with beta blockers in several large-scale studies (e.g., Medical Research Council).[1] Prevention of coronary events is even less marked, especially with the use of thiazide diuretics. Equivocal results with beta blockers and other antisympathetic agents may be related to adverse effects on serum lipids, hemodynamics, or other factors induced by the agents used. In the Medical Research Council trial, coronary events were reduced in nonsmoking males on beta blockers but actually increased in smokers, both male and female.[1]

Increased age is perhaps the principal "risk factor" for the occurrence of stroke and coronary events, especially in women. Since age is irreversible, it is hardly justifiable to reduce enjoyment of one's remaining years for questionable benefit of lowered blood pressure. Treatment should certainly be avoided or terminated if it interferes with an individual's ability to function independently, if it poses a high risk of life-threatening side effects, or if it interferes with treatment for more acute conditions.

Course of Treatment

Who Should be Treated

Aggressive treatment may be justified for males manifesting severe hypertension at any age unless contraindicated; for females and males postinfarction who do not show a spontaneous drop in blood pressure; for males and females poststroke; for males with moderate hypertension at high risk (especially if they have left ventricular hypertrophy or glucose intolerance); for diabetic females with mild to severe hypertension, especially if they are black and/or under 60.

Less aggressive treatment may be justified for other males with mild-to-moderate blood pressure; for females over 60 with mean blood pressure over 120 mmHg; for other postmenopausal females deemed at high risk.

Evaluation

Simply determining blood pressure at rest is not sufficient to judge the efficacy of antihypertensive treatment. The impedance testing we use (see Chapter 8) is desirable to indicate whether the medication is normalizing all parts of the blood pressure equation, not just the blood pressure. That is, since Blood Pressure = Cardiac Output × Total Systemic Resistance, cardiac output and total systemic resistance must be normalized as well. Blood pressure readings should also be taken during mental stress. We have found that even with hypotensive medication, a patient may still have an untoward reactivity in response to mental stress. As is explained in Chapter 10 (Ambulatory Monitoring), this is important, because this accurately predicts the average daily blood pressure, which, in turn, is predictive of future target organ damage such as left ventricular hypertrophy.[6]

Follow-up for side effects should include questions on any change in other medications perhaps prescribed by others, including nonprescription drugs. Interactions can often alter the effectiveness and side effects of antihypertensive drugs. Measurement of blood pressure, standing as well as seated, is most advisable to reveal postural hypotension.

Step-Down Therapy

After blood pressure has been maintained at the desired level for six months or more, "step-down" therapy can be attempted. The idea is to permit the patient to use the minimum dosage needed whenever possible. Finnerty[7] was able to reduce the dosage or to eliminate one of two drugs in 42 patients of a group of 51 who had been treated for moderately severe and severe hypertension for 6 months. Another group of 67 patients with diastolic blood pressure 92-104 mmHg and a high level of risk factors were stepped-down from 50 mg of chlorthalidone per day after six months of control (DBP < 85 mmHg). The dosage was reduced to 25 mg, then after 3 months to 12.5 mg, then in 3 months to zero unless the diastolic blood pressure increased above 85 mmHg. The medication was thus discontinued for 59 patients, and at 24 months 38 of these still were maintaining their diastolic blood pressure under 85 mmHg. After 57 months, 36 of the 67 remained in good control without therapy; of those who restarted therapy, only 28 were followed up at 57 months and all but two of these were being maintained on reduced dosage.[8] Others have reported similar success. Alderman et al[9] found that more than two thirds of 66 patients deemed suitable for step-down therapy were able to maintain normal pressure without drugs for over a year, including 7 of 8 patients with higher initial pressures (SBP at least 180 and/or DBP at least 105). They also noted that patients maintained successfully for a year without drugs rarely had an increase in mean blood pressure the second year.[9] In the Framingham study, 95 (8%) of those identified as hypertensive were observed to maintain normal blood pressure without medication for several years. Although all eventually became hypertensive over a 14-year period, 11 of the 95 maintained good control without medication for at least four years.[10] In a controlled study of nutritional therapy, 5% of those without any special nutritional therapy maintained normal blood pressures for four years without medication, and 39% of those undergoing nutritional intervention (weight-loss, reduced sodium intake, reduced alcohol intake) remained normotensive for four years.[11]

Pharmacologic Agents

Output Hypertensives

Output hypertensives are generally young or in the early stage of hypertension. If behavioral therapy is not effective, output hypertensives generally will respond to beta-adrenergic blocking agents.

Beta-adrenergic Blocking Agents

Beta-adrenergic blocking agents reduce cardiac output and also inhibit renin release from the kidney. Nonspecific beta blockers (β_1 and β_2 inhibition) are propanolol, timolol, and nadolol. Pindolol is also nonselective but with intrinsic sympathomimetic action (ISA). This is manifested by a smaller reduction in the resting heart rate than is seen with other beta blockers lacking ISA. Cardioselective β_1 inhibitors include atenolol, metoprolol, and acebutolol. An agent that combines both beta- and alpha-blocking properties is labetalol.

Contraindications for using beta-adrenergic blocking agents are asthma, broncho-obstructive lung disease, congestive heart failure, and second or third degree heart block. They are not advisable for diabetics because they may blunt symptoms of hypoglycemia.[12] If they must be used for a diabetic, the cardioselective agents are preferable.

Beta blockers or other sympatholytic drugs may be appropriate for high-renin essential hypertension (which is accompanied by high cardiac output[13] and occurs mainly in whites under 40); alcohol-withdrawal hypertension; orthostatic hypertension; postmyocardial infarction; ventricular ectopy; increased beta-adrenergic responsiveness.[14] They have been found to reduce the incidence of reinfarction in post MI patients.

Combined Hypertensives

The combination of increased output and increased resistance occurs as blood vessels thicken in response to the increased output. Labetalol, which combines both beta- and alpha-blocking properties, is a good choice for most combined hypertensives. Alternatively, a beta blocker can be combined with the alpha blocker prazosin or another vasodilating agent.

Vasoconstrictive Hypertensives

In older persons or chronic hypertensives, the vasoconstrictive type of hypertension is more prevalent. Many agents with different modes of action are now available, so that we no longer rely mainly on diuretics which have several adverse consequences.

α_1 Blockers

The α_1 blocker prazosin is useful for a wide variety of patients. Prazosin does not have adverse effects on plasma lipids or glucose tolerance and maintains normal cardiac output and renal blood flow. It has been used successfully in patients with impaired renal function, bronchospasm, diabetes mellitus, and other abnormalities.[15] It is effective in young and old, white and black, and high- or low-renin hypertensives. Unlike beta blockers, it does not reduce the heart rate or attenuate the cardiac output increase with exercise. Sodium retention is not a major problem with prazosin.[16] Diabetics may demonstrate improvement in glucose tolerance tests.[17]

A further advantage for the elderly is the fact that this agent does not impair cerebral blood flow. This is important because many antihypertensive agents have been found to impair central nervous system function in the elderly[18] leading to confusion or even delirium.

Diabetic men reportedly have less sexual dysfunction with prazosin than with agents such as methyldopa or clonidine.[19]

The main side effects of this agent are dizziness, vertigo, weakness and headache, but they are generally transient or tolerable.[20] They are less bothersome if the medication is taken at bedtime.[21]

Severe hypotension or syncope can occur with the first dose and appropriate precautions should be taken. This is not a problem with later doses, however.

Slow Channel Calcium-Entry Blocking Agents

The calcium-entry blockers such as diltiazem, verapamil, and nifedipine have a direct dilating effect on the arterial wall and have some venodilator effects as well. They thus increase both coronary and cerebral blood flow.[22] All are effective antihypertensive agents generally without undesirable metabolic side effects. They maintain blood flow to the kidneys, brain, and heart and cause less fluid retention than other vasodilators.[22] They are more effective in low- rather than high-renin hypertensives.[23] They are all able to reduce blood pressure by lowering total peripheral resistance in mild, moderate, and severe hypertension. Diltiazem, however, has the advantage of lowering heart rate and myocardial oxygen consumption.[24] Nifedipine has been used frequently for control of severe hypertension, both acutely (sublingually) and chronically.[22]

At this writing verapamil is the only one approved by the FDA for antihypertensive therapy, although it seems likely that others soon will be approved as well. Verapamil can be used in patients with chronic obstructive pulmonary disease, asthma, renal failure, congestive heart failure, ischemic heart disease, and peripheral vascular disease. Thus it may be particularly suitable for elderly hypertensives with concomitant conditions, although long-term experience is lacking. It does not cause postural hypotension, sedation or depression.[25] Rebound hypertension on cessation has not been seen with the calcium blockers.

The effects of calcium-entry blockers on glucose metabolism seem to be variable. Therefore careful monitoring is required in treating diabetics.[22]

One of the disadvantages of these drugs is the comparative difficulty in titration of the dosage.

Contraindications are severe left ventricular dysfunction, sick sinus syndrome, second- or third-degree atrioventricular block, and hypotension. Among the common side effects are pedal edema (0.6% to 10% of patients on nifedipine), headache and flushing. These occur more frequently with nifedipine than with verapamil and diltiazem.[22] The most common side effect of verapamil is constipation.

Angiotensin-Converting Enzyme (ACE) Inhibitors

Captopril and enalapril are specific competitive inhibitors of angiotensin I converting enzyme (ACE). This enzyme is responsible for the conversion of angiotensin I, a relatively inactive substance, to angiotensin II, a potent endogenous vasoconstrictor. These agents are especially recommended for patients with high-renin hypertension. They are less effective in patients over 40 than in younger hypertensives.[26]

An abrupt fall in blood pressure and rise in plasma-renin-activity levels in response to a single dose of captopril are characteristics of renovascular hypertension.

In a study evaluating effects on quality of life, captopril was deemed to relate to more favorable changes than methyldopa or propranolol.[27]

Food interferes with the availability of captopril, so it must be taken on an empty stomach two or three times daily.[28]

Side effects of captopril include dermatitis and hyperkalemia in patients with renal insufficiency. It has also been found to cause proteinuria and should not be used for patients with impaired kidney function or stenosis of a renal artery.[29] Therefore careful evaluation of renal function is important, especially for diabetics, before using this agent. It may impair the sense of taste leading to anorexia in some patients and possibly interfering with diabetic control. Another concern for diabetics is that captopril can cause a false-positive urine test for acetone.[17] When mean daily doses of captopril are no higher than 324 mg per day, the incidence of side effects is low.[30] Allergic reactions are in the range of 6% to 10 percent and neutropenia (the most severe side effect) is about 0.3 percent.[28] Halitosis, however, is rather common and this seemingly minor problem can devastate a patient's social life.

Enalapril is a newer type of ACE inhibitor with a different chemical structure and longer duration of action than captopril. In contrast to captopril, therapy with this agent is believed to be beneficial to patients with renal parenchymal disease and renovascular hypertension.[31]

The incidence of side effects, such as skin rash and taste disturbances, are much lower with enalapril than with captopril, and proteinuria has not been reported in patients treated with it.[30] Food does not interfere with the bioavailability of enalapril as it does with captopril. Both enalapril and captopril treatment have caused coughing and wheezing to a distressing degree in a few patients.[32]

Enalapril is effective as monotherapy in 55% to 66% of patients and addition of a diuretic increases its effectiveness to 85% to 95%. This combination is beneficial in that the two agents potentiate each other and enalapril protects against excessive loss of potassium and magnesium from the diuretic action. Enalapril has been effective in patients with low and normal renin as well as in high-renin hypertensives. It has been used in patients with mild, moderate, and severe hypertension; with concurrent conditions including bronchial asthma, diabetes mellitus, coronary insufficiency, and chronic renal failure.[28]

Additional Sympatholytics

Besides the alpha- and beta-adrenergic blocking agents, the adrenergic inhibitors include the central alpha-adrenergic agonists such as methyldopa and clonidine; and agents acting on postganglionic nerve endings such as reserpine and guanethidine. These agents reduce the adrenergic input to the heart, blood vessels, and kidneys. They reduce the total systemic resistance by reducing the smooth muscle tone of arterials. The undesirable side effects of these drugs are orthostatic hypotension and sexual dysfunction.

Methyldopa causes drowsiness but still may be preferable for an elderly person since it has minimal renal effects and rarely causes postural hypotension, especially if given in small doses two or three times a day. Clonidine also can be used in the elderly, but the possibility of noncompliance must be considered since sudden withdrawal can result in a sharp rise in blood pressure.[29] Guanfacine, which is longer-acting than clonidine, is less likely to cause withdrawal reactions.[21] It also has the advantage of reducing serum cholesterol levels.[33] Guanfacine has been effective in patients with congestive heart failure, diabetes, and renal dysfunction. Principal side effects are dry mouth, tiredness, and constipation.[34]

Reserpine, which has been in use a long time, is now generally avoided because it can lead to severe depression in some patients. In small doses (e.g., 0.1 mg per day) side effects are minimal, although over time, postural hypotension can develop.[29]

Guanethidine is used primarily for severe hypertension.[29] This drug is also generally avoided because of its high rate of side effects, especially orthostatic hypotension.

Vasodilators

Vasodilators such as hydralazine, minoxidil, and diazoxide produce relaxation of vascular smooth muscle with reduction of total systemic resistance. They may increase cardiac output if reflex cardiac stimulation is intact, with palpitations and tachycardia as side effects. They may also induce fluid retention.

Because it maintains renal flow, hydralazine has been used in patients with renal failure.[14]

Large doses of hydralazine may produce a lupus erythematosus syndrome. Minoxidil also can have serious side effects, and is indicated only in the treatment of severe hypertension refractory to other medications. Diazoxide is an injectable nondiuretic benzodiathiazine for short-term emergency treatment of malignant hypertension. Sodium nitroprusside used only as an infusion with sterile 5% dextrose in water is another agent for emergency treatment of hypertensive crises.

Indapamide is a thiazidelike agent that in subdiuretic doses may act as a vasodilator.

Diuretics

When there are evidences of sodium and water retention in the mechanism of hypertension, diuresis is the appropriate measure for lowering blood pressure. Diuretics inhibit sodium reabsorption: thiazides (such as hydrochlorothiazide) in the proximal and distal tubule, furosamide acting in the countermultiplier system of loop of Henle, and the potassium-sparing agents (spironolactone, triamterene, and amiloride) in the distal tubule.

Because these agents are well tolerated by most patients, are inexpensive and are generally effective as monotherapy, they may be preferable where compliance or cost are major considerations. (Note that the potassium-sparing diuretics are rarely used alone.)

Diuretics are particularly useful for blacks, the obese, and patients with congestive heart failure. If there is evidence of hypokalemia, a low-sodium diet or a combination of a thiazide and a potassium-sparing diuretic agent is preferable to adding a potassium supplement.[35] Although diuretics have been used by both type I and type II diabetics under careful supervision,[12] they are far less acceptable for diabetic patients.

Diuretics have undesirable effects that include hypokalemia, hyperuricemia, hyperglycemia, and hyperlipidemia. Thiazides have reportedly had a diabetogenic effect in some cases particularly when used in the higher doses, and they may increase the risk of coronary events among women who smoke.[1] The MRFIT study[36] also showed an apparent increase in mortality with treatment of patients who had electrocardiographic abnormalities as well as hypertension. However, diuretics have been used as first-step therapy alone and in conjunction with other antihypertensives in a great many patients, generally without major adverse effects. Since they are well known and are relatively inexpensive, they are still the most popular choice of most clinicians. If their use is not contraindicated for a particular patient and if the patient is monitored for metabolic effects, they can provide satisfactory treatment. For persons with normal renal function, combinations with the potassium-sparing ones may be preferable. The tendency now is to use lower dosages of the diuretics than in the past (25 to 50 mg of hydrochlorthiazide or equivalent) since it has been determined that this is the range of maximal effectiveness. Dose-related side effects are therefore fewer in number.[37]

Elderly persons should be started at very low doses and the distal tubular diuretics are preferable. The Hypertension Detection and Follow-Up Program[38] showed the benefit of diuretic treatment in reduced stroke mortality among treated persons 60 to 69 years of age who had both diastolic (DBP at least 90) and systolic hypertension. Although treatment of isolated systolic hypertension is somewhat controversial, the Langfords[39] suggest treating it if the mean blood pressure is at least 120 mmHg for several readings over a period of months. Elderly persons, however, must be frequently monitored for side effects and metabolic changes especially for hypokalemia and hyponatremia. The risk of diuretic-induced hyponatremia is greatest in aged females below average body weight or with a tendency to dehydration.[40]

References

1. Medical Research Council Working Party. MRC trial of treatment of mild hypertension: principal results. Br Med J 291:97–104, 1985.
2. Hulka BS, Cassel JC, Lawrence LK, et al. Communications, compliance and concordance between physicians and patients with prescribed medication. Am J Public Health 66:847–853, 1976.
3. Moser M. Treating hypertension: a review of clinical trials. Am J Med 81(suppl 6C):25–32, 1986.
4. Forsyth RA. Coronary heart disease in treated hypertensive patients and risk-matched normotensive control subjects. Am Heart J 108:305–310, 1984.
5. Dollery CT. Risk predictors, risk indicators, and benefit factors in hypertension. Am J Med 82(suppl 1A):2–8, 1987.
6. Perloff D, Sokolow M, Cowan R. The prognostic value of ambulatory blood pressures. JAMA 249:2792–2798, 1983.
7. Finnerty FA Jr. Step-down treatment of mild systemic hypertension. Am J Cardiol 53:1304–1307, 1984.
8. Finnerty FA. Step-down therapy in hypertension: its importance in long-term management. JAMA 246:2593–2596, 1981.
9. Alderman MH, Davis TK, Gerber LM, et al. Antihypertensive drug therapy withdrawal in a general population. Arch Intern Med 146:1309–1311, 1986.
10. Dannenberg AL, Kannel WB. Remission of hypertension. The 'natural' history of blood pressure treatment in the Framingham study. JAMA 257:1477–1483, 1987.
11. Stamler R, Stamler J, Grimm R, et al. Nutritional therapy for high blood pressure: final report of a four-year randomized controlled trial—The Hypertension Control Program. JAMA 257:1484–1491, 1987.

12. Christlieb AR. Treating hypertension in the patient with diabetes mellitus. Clin North Am 66(6):1373–1388, 1982.
13. Dustan HP. Pathophysiology of hypertension. In: Hurst JW (ed), The Heart, Sixth Edition. McGraw-Hill, New York, 1986. pp 1038–1048.
14. Wollam GL, Hall WD. Treatment of systemic hypertension. In: Hurst JW (ed), The Heart, Sixth Edition. McGraw-Hill, New York, 1986, pp 1071–1090.
15. Okun R. Effectiveness of prazosin as initial antihypertensive therapy. Am J Cardiol 51:644–650, 1983.
16. Dzau VJ. Evolution of the clinical management of hypertension: emerging role of "specific" vasodilators as initial therapy. Am J Med 82(suppl 1A):36–43, 1987.
17. Cherner R. Antihypertensive agents & diabetes: Side effects that demand careful consideration. Consultant 27(2):22–34, 1987.
18. Ram CVS, Meese R, Kaplan NM, et al. Antihypertensive therapy in the elderly: effects on blood pressure and cerebral blood flow. Am J Med 82(suppl 1A):53–57, 1987.
19. Lipson LG. Special problems: treatment of hypertension in the patient with diabetes mellitus. Arch Intern Med 144:1829–1831, 1984.
20. Kincaid-Smith PS. Alpha blockade: an overview of efficacy data. Am J Med 82(suppl 1A):21–25, 1987.
21. Reid JL. Alpha-adrenergic receptors and blood pressure control. Am J Cardiol 57:6E–12E, 1986.
22. Halperin AK, Cubeddu LX. The role of calcium channel blockers in the treatment of hypertension. Am Heart J 111:363 382, 1986.
23. Messerli FH, Garavaglia GE. Cardiodynamics of hypertension: a guide to selection of therapy. J Clin Hypertens 3:100S–108S, 1986.
24. Schulte KL, Meyer-Sabellek, WA, Haertenberger A, et al. Antihypertensive and metabolic effects of diltiazem and nifedipine. Hypertension 8:859 865, 1986.
25. Ben-Ishay D, Leibel B, Stessman J. Calcium channel blockers in the management of hypertension in the elderly. Am J Med 81(suppl 6A):30–34, 1986.
26. Epstein M. Targeting antihypertensive therapy to the individual patient. J Clin Hypertension 2(3 Suppl):62S–71S, 1986.
27. Croog SH, Levine S, Testa MA, et al. The effects of antihypertensive therapy on the quality of life. N Engl J Med 314:1657–1664, 1986.
28. Gavras I, Gavras H. Clinical utility of angiotensin converting enzyme inhibitors in hypertension. Am J Med 81(suppl 4C):28–31, 1986.
29. Shapiro AP, McDonald RH Jr. Renal effects of antihypertensive drugs in the elderly. Geriatric Medicine Today 5(1):59–64, 1986.
30. Irvin JD, Viau JM. Safety profiles of the angiotensin converting enzyme inhibitors captopril and enalapril. Am J Med 81(suppl 4C):46–50, 1986.
31. Bauer JH, Reams GP. Renal effects of angiotensin converting enzyme inhibitors in hypertension. Am J Med 81(suppl 4C):19–27, 1986.
32. Semple PF, Herd GW. Cough and wheeze caused by inhibitors of angiotensin-converting enzyme. New Engl J Med 314:61, 1986 (letter).

33. Hauger-Klevene JH, Balossi EC, Scornavacchi JC. Effects of guanfacine on growth hormone, prolactin, renin, lipoproteins and glucose in essential hypertension. Am J Cardiol 57:27E–31E, 1986.

34. Jerie P. Long-term evaluations of therapeutic efficacy and safety of guanfacine. Am J Cardiol 57:55E–59E, 1986.

35. Gifford RW Jr. Role of diuretics in treatment of essential hypertension. Am J Cardiol 58:15A–17A, 1986.

36. Multiple Risk Factor Intervention Trial Research Group. Baseline rest electrocardiographic abnormalities, antihypertensive treatment and mortality in the multiple risk factor intervention trial. Am J Cardiol 55:1–15, 1985.

37. Gifford R. Discussion II. Am J Med 81(suppl 6C):51, 1986.

38. Hypertension Detection and Follow-up Program Cooperative Group: five-year findings of the hypertension detection and follow-up program. III. Reduction in stroke incidence among persons with high blood pressure. JAMA 247:633–638, 1982.

39. Langford HG, Langford MJ. Systolic hypertension in the elderly. Geriatric Med Today 4(9):47–52, 1985.

40. Ayus JC. Diuretic-induced hyponatremia. Arch Intern Med 146:1295–1296, 1986 (Editorial).

Chapter 14

Rehabilitation

Robert S. Eliot
David R. Long
Jeffrey L. Boone

Introduction

The aim of cardiovascular rehabilitation is to improve the quality of life for cardiac patients to permit them to function at the highest level compatible with the extent of their disease,[1] and to reduce future morbidity through proper treatment and risk factor reduction. This definition highlights the altruistic ideals of the program. However, all too often, physicians become ensnared in a "technology trap" which deemphasizes the most important part of this definition—*the Quality of Life*. Great care and attention are placed on the pharmacology and the medical aspects of cardiac rehabilitation, but pertinent psychological issues of sexuality, identity, employability, and attitude are not adequately addressed. Since physicians play lead roles either as program directors of cardiac rehabilitation or as primary care physicians, they need to coordinate closely with the rehabilitation team to improve all aspects of therapy that impact on a patient's quality of life.

It is our hope that this chapter will increase awareness of the importance of physician support for the psychosocial and behavioral aspects of cardiac rehabilitation. Certainly we do not want to de-emphasize the need for sophisticated medical technology in rehabilitation. Instead, we propose a tighter bond between medical and behavioral

From: Eliot, RS: *Stress and the Heart: Mechanisms, Measurements and Management.* Mount Kisco, NY, Futura Publishing Company, Inc., © 1988.

management in treating the cardiovascular patient. Perhaps then we shall see a greater return to gainful employment and high quality, productive lives.

In the Hospital

Rehabilitation starts as soon as the patient has been identified as a victim of MI, sudden death, or as a candidate for cardiac surgery. As Norman Cousins emphasized in his book *The Healing Heart*,[2] relief from panic is the first requirement for a heart-attack victim. Patients anticipating surgery need reassurance too, and also information on what to expect in the hospital. Although this seems obvious, by-pass patients frequently express their dissatisfaction with preoperative information. Their anger stems from failure to be told about the endotracheal tube, which is uncomfortable and prevents talking, and restrictions from other postoperative paraphernalia and procedures.[3] Also, they should be forewarned of postoperative depression and various types of "normal" pains and discomforts and be reassured as to their meaning and temporary nature. While optimistic deniers may not want such information, others may need it to allay overanxiety. The amount of information to be supplied is a clinical "judgment call" in each case. The physician as the principal figure in the entire hospitalization too often neglects the leadership role in dealing with behavioral issues that may significantly affect outcome.

The CCU

In the hospital, nurses play a major role in determining the mental state of their patients and thus the rate of their recovery. The mechanistic aspects of the ICU or CCU, the impersonal concern with technical equipment and numbers, all tend to make the patient feel dehumanized, helpless, and hopeless. The touch of a hand or a few words of reassurance addressed directly to him/her is calming and restores hope.

Besides the stress of the illness, the unfamiliar surroundings, the threat of death, and the discomfort of monitoring equipment add to the patient's anxiety. The first step then must be to provide comfort in the form of human contact and to explain the machinery and protocol of the CCU. Since patients may be anxious and somewhat confused and disoriented, explanations may have to be repeated several times. Anxiolytic agents are recommended for many patients, especially those who show heightened reactions to stresses such as physicians on rounds, alarm bells, etc.[4]

Some patients use denial to cope with their fear. Those who reject the reality of their illness may balk at the necessary treatment. However, those who accept the reality of the illness but deny its seriousness actually seem to have a better prognosis,[5] at least in the acute phase. Thus total elimination of denial at this stage is unnecessary and unwise. Later, one must deal with reality.

Many patients dislike being among the sick. The hospital situation in general tends to make one feel helpless, with loss of control and loss of identity; in addition, a brush with death and the fear of serious consequences from the heart condition can damage the patient's self-esteem. Thus, the three stress factors that are worst for health—loss of control, identity, and self-esteem—are present and must be overcome. Adequate pain medication postoperatively and anxiolytics, where indicated, can speed recovery.

One back-handed but effective way to reassure MI patients on their second day in the CCU is to say, "You know, more people die from a heart attack during the first 24 hours than during the next 5 years. You've made it through the crucial first day, so let's start planning for the next 5 years."

The combination of strange surroundings, illness, medications, and disturbed sleep leads to "CCU psychosis" in a large number of patients. This is especially likely for elderly infarct patients who suddenly and unexpectedly find themselves immobilized in frightening surroundings. Dr. Boone tells the story of an independent and muscular 90-year-old lumberjack who woke up in the CCU after a slight MI. Not understanding what had happened or where he was, he repeatedly ripped out the urinary catheters and broke out of restraints. The more extreme the measures tried by the medical staff, the more his mental state worsened, and some staff members were sure he was hopelessly psychotic. When the decision was finally reached (mainly out of desperation) to treat the fellow at home, his mental state returned to normal and his recovery continued uneventfully. Although he showed some signs of senility over the next three years, he definitely was not psychotic.

Patients are less likely to become disoriented if there are windows and clocks to indicate time of day, and if they are talked *to* rather than *about* even if they are unable to reply. We strongly advocate a role for the family physician in the CCU. The person who has just had an MI feels as though he/she has been cut off from everything—even life itself. It reassures the patient to see the one physician who knows him as a human being. The more technically oriented cardiologists may seem to be more concerned with the machines to which the patients are attached than to the human beings they are monitoring. The family physician also is better able to relay information to the family members who generally feel more comfortable discussing their concerns with him/her than with the cardiologist.

The CCU should be set up to provide some privacy to the individuals. Witnessing the death or near-death of a patient in the next bed is not conducive to psychological tranquility!

For the heart attack patient, an important question to be faced in the CCU is "Why now?" The factors that led to or were associated with the event must be faced in order to speed recovery, return the patient to gainful life, and prevent recurrence.

Ideally, the hospital rehabilitation program will include psychological evaluation and counseling and educational material specific for that particular patient and spouse. Booklets describing what to expect in the hospital and explaining the phases of recovery are desirable. People may not comprehend what is told to them while they are overwrought and thus may absorb the information better when they read it at a calmer moment. However, someone must take the time to answer questions about the material and to individualize the advice to the particular case. Except for those few patients who enjoy the role of an invalid, it is restorative to learn that in a few weeks they can resume sexual activity, most other normal physical activity and, in the majority of cases, return to work. Since financial strains are often a major problem to these patients, it can be a great relief if they can be assured that most likely they will be able to return to productivity in a relatively short time.

At some period, depression sets in. This may occur as early as three to five days after MI or surgery, or appear later after the patient has left the hospital. This has been likened to the mourning for a loss: in this case a sense of lost potential or lost physical ability.[5] Generally, the depression is transient and talking about his/her concerns may be the best treatment. The patient needs reassurance that weakness is to be expected during recuperation. The patient should also be given the opportunity to discuss financial and domestic problems, which often top the list of patient concerns.

A few patients will become angry and uncooperative. This may be a response to feeling isolated and helpless. If a doctor or nurse takes the time to listen to the patient's complaints and to explain the rationale for procedures and treatments, the patient can often be persuaded to cooperate.

Although transfer out of the CCU is generally regarded as a positive sign by patients, they may also experience some anxiety from the reduced protective surveillance and separation from familiar surroundings and personnel. They can be reassured and gain a feeling of continuity if they are shown the new surroundings and meet one or more of the staff who will be attending them before the move is made.

Post-CCU Hospital Stay

Since prolonged bed rest causes weakening, an early effort to reduce muscular deconditioning is important. Mild exercises to improve range of motion for arms and legs can be started in the acute care unit. Then short walks can be instituted and gradually increased in duration. Patients are encouraged by each increase in the time and/or distance they can walk before becoming fatigued.

The educational phase of rehabilitation should start immediately after transfer from the CCU. Those who feel they have had a brush with death are particularly amenable to suggestions for behavioral change such as smoking cessation, diet modification, and relaxation therapy. This is the "golden moment" for behavioral change. Some hospitals have daily sessions for patients (often open to spouses and friends) with a different topic each day presented by the appropriate member of the rehabilitation team. Other hospitals individualize the education and do not include the spouse; they feel the patient may hesitate to discuss some sensitive subjects in the presence of others, including the spouse. Probably a combination of both is ideal. Group therapy reinforces the benefits of "one-on-one", in our experience. It adds an immeasureable therapeutic dimension of mutual support and esprit de "coeur."

Authoritative information can dispel concerns caused by harmful "myths" about cardiac conditions and aid in adaptive coping by both patients and family.

As Anderson[6] has pointed out, "The kinds of information that contribute to adaptive coping include basic information about the nature and extent of their cardiac condition, explanations of their symptoms in terms of their cardiac condition, adequate rationales for recommended behavioral changes (e.g., Why is smoking detrimental to your heart?), explanations of the purpose of cardiac medications and of their common side effects, and explanations of expected emotional responses to their cardiac status. . . . Appropriate information contributes to adaptive coping by correcting unrealistic appraisals of threat, by reducing uncertainty and thus increasing the sense of control, and by suggesting new (more appropriate) coping strategies."

Pre-discharge

Pre-discharge counseling includes a review of the necessary restrictions on activity and diet, medication schedule, and desired behavioral modifications. In addition, the major stressors should be discussed. Arrangements can then be made for special needs such as nursing or household help, financial aid, etc. Employment counseling is important for those who may need to make changes in their occupation or who have previously been too disabled to work and have lost confidence in themselves. Sexual matters are another major concern that should be discussed.

Enrollment in a formal rehabilitation program is desirable but may not be feasible for all patients. In that case, a program of daily exercise and increasing physical activity can be outlined. The behavioral components can be supplemented with audio and video tapes, for example. An exercise test (low-level treadmill test) is frequently administered to post-MI or postsurgical patients to determine the "exercise prescription." This is described more fully in Chapter 9 (Treadmill Testing and Exercise Prescription). Those who do well on the exercise test gain self-confidence and greater self-efficacy. For those less fortunate, the physician should emphasize the benefits of the indicated therapeutic options.

For surgical patients, walking programs can usually be accomplished, but arduous activity must be delayed until the sternotomy is healed.

Posthospital Rehabilitation

Depression

As mentioned earlier, the patient may become depressed after returning home, even if there were no signs during hospitalization. The symptoms may be manifested by "somatization" with such physical signs as pain and fatigue instead of or in addition to mental ones.

If the physician is made aware of the depression, he/she can reassure the patient that such feelings are common and usually pass in a short time. If the patient is taking medications that tend to aggravate depression (beta blockers, for instance, or certain antihypertensives), modifications in treatment should be considered. No other therapy may be necessary but close follow-up is required. Antidepressant medication or professional psychiatric care may be indicated in some cases. Loss of appetite, insomnia, a feeling of isolation, and general apathy are among the signs that may indicate serious depression.[5]

Activities associated with a rehabilitation program tend to help resolve transient depression. Patients who are deemed ineligible for an exercise program may be the ones needing more psychologic counseling. The physician and/or counselor can introduce such patients to stress management techniques and other beneficial measures to help them feel they are again in control of their lives.

Spouse and Family

The concerns of the spouse should also be considered. Even with an in-hospital education program and a discharge pamphlet of information, spouses may not be prepared for the actual problems of convalescence. They may understand dietary needs, for instance, but not know how to apply them to the daily menu. They may disagree with the patient on whether specific activities are within permitted physical guidelines—especially driving a car and sexual activities. The spouse may also express concern because of a patient's overdependence or depression.[7]

The patient's family or significant other needs education and support to deal with the stress of the situation which usually involves heightened responsibilities as well as the problem of dealing with an agitated patient. The crisis situation of the heart attack or the cardiac surgery very frequently unleashes previously suppressed emotional problems. There is often much unexpressed anger on the part of the spouse. This stems from a variety of often unapparent causes, such as anger with regard to separation and the threat of dying when "we haven't really lived yet," financial concerns for maintaining the lifestyle, guilt that marital discord may have been a contributing factor, or irritation when a divorce is delayed.

If surgery is prescribed, family members, as well as patients will want to know what to expect—how long the hospitalization will be, what are the expected reactions to the surgery and medication, what care will be needed at home, etc. If they are allowed to visit in the intensive care area, they should be forewarned that patients often do not recognize their visitors.[8]

The role changes and stresses resulting from a coronary event can cause emotional problems up to two years later, and may have an adverse effect on the marriage.[9]

Private counseling sessions for individual couples may be advisable to aid adjustments, especially if the couple find it difficult to communicate their concerns to each other.

Educational sessions and support groups for spouses can help to ease the problems they face. The sessions can explain the course of the disease and how to go about making the necessary lifestyle changes that will reduce the patients' risks and enhance their compliance with prescribed treatment. It should also include information on how the spouses themselves can cope with their added responsibilities and their anxieties about the patient's health and mood, and how to avoid relegating the patient to a permanent sick role.

Dracup et al[9] noted that the couples participating in group sessions benefited from the shared experience of others and the mutual concern and understanding of the group members.

Having spouses participate in the exercise classes with the patients or enabling the spouses to witness the treadmill testing has been found to reassure them as to the patients' physical capabilities.[10] Learning CPR also gives family members a better sense of control and helps allay their anxiety, but in some cases the patients may become more anxious.[11]

Sexual Concerns

Although sexual functioning is a major concern for most cardiac patients, few feel free to discuss this sensitive subject with their physicians or surgeons, and very few physicians provide the needed information voluntarily. This is especially true of those over 50 (both patients and physicians) who grew up in a more sexually conservative era. Physicians should try to overcome this reticence and offer information in an objective, nonthreatening fashion that will allay fears and anxiety. The chapter on sexual counseling offers suggestions on how this can be done.

Resumption of sexual activity may be very important in the marital relationship during the stressful readjustment period. It is a common misconception that sexual activity is too strenuous. Actually it has been found that for men the energy expenditure is only 5 METs at orgasm and 3.7 METs before and after orgasm, that is, heart rate of about 110 to 120 beats per minute at the peak.[12] Any patient able to climb a flight of stairs briskly should be capable of this degree of activity. However, some researchers have reported dysrhythmias during intercourse in patients monitored by ECG. These are less likely to occur with a familiar partner, such as the spouse, than in an extramarital adventure.[13]

Angina during intercourse can be devastating to a patient; therefore, it may be advisable for some patients to use nitroglycerin prior to sexual activity, particularly before the first attempt after hospitalization. Shine[14] recommends that patients learn to administer the medication before discharge to relieve anxiety about the medication itself.

While a few individuals may find a cardiac event a convenient excuse to retreat from undesired sexual activity, most patients do want to have a normal sex life. According to Papadopoulos,[15] more post-CABG patients than post-MI patients resume sex, develop fewer symptoms in relation to it, and have intercourse more often. This may be due to the fact that some who had suffered angina before are now able to enjoy sex without pain. However, some patients with a good surgical result show no improvement in sexual functioning, and the patient (or the couple) may need the help of a psychologist to find the source of the difficulty.

Exercise

Enrollment in a formal outpatient rehabilitation program that is a continuation of the hospital program is probably ideal and should be encouraged. Prolonged inactivity increases the patients deconditioning and their feelings of weakness and helplessness which in turn may add to their anxiety. Participation in exercise programs can help patients feel they are taking control, and they gain psychosocial support as well as physical conditioning. If the patient cannot get to a rehabilitation center, home therapy may be possible. A study by Miller et al[16] demonstrated that carefully selected low-risk patients post-MI could achieve increases in functional capacity through home training comparable to the results of group training. Their patients used portable heart rate monitors and were checked by telephone twice weekly.

However, as with many other special medical conditions, other patients who have been through the experience can provide meaningful psychosocial support. Thus the rehabilitation group itself offers helpful support as there is empathy among the members, and they encourage each other.

The program should be in a supervised setting with equipment available for monitoring those most at risk and for handling cardiac emergencies. Recommended equipment includes a defibrillator and other emergency medical equipment, radio telemetry units for those patients whose cardiac condition requires constant monitoring, electrocardiographic recorders, exercise bicycles, arm ergometers, motor-driven treadmill, and other exercise equipment.

In the experience of such cardiac rehabilitation programs, the risk is minimal. One review of 30 programs[17] estimated that there was one event per 33,000 hours of exercise, and one death per 120,000 patient hours. Among groups with CAD in Seattle, approximately one episode of cardiac arrest occurred per 10,400 hours of exercise. Programs with continuous ECG monitoring report fewer complications than those without it. Since most events occur in the warm-up and post-training periods, supervision at these times is especially important. Those most at risk have been characterized as those who exceed their prescribed target heart rates and those who show significant ST depression persisting more than one minute into recovery after exercise testing.

In general, the goals of rehabilitation with regard to reduction of risk factors, training in stress management, and increase in cardiovascular fitness are similar to those of preventive programs. The exercise portion must be carefully individualized and monitored. Attention must be given to the psychological aspects of rehabilitation to minimize depression and anxiety and maximize compliance. The key to success lies with the personnel—how they understand the goals of rehabilitation and relate to the individual patient.

Group learning sessions with formal lectures are important, but almost everyone also requires one-on-one counseling for individual problems. The total program must be supervised by an experienced physician, and hopefully all personnel will have basic training and will demonstrate good judgment and empathy.

For the first two weeks of exercise the patient is monitored by means of telemetry. The aim is to keep the level of exertion within 5 beats/min of the target heart rate. Evidence of ST depression, dysrhythmia, ectopic beats, etc. warrant intervention. Target heart rate initially is regulated by the patient's demonstrated ability on the entry treadmill examination. We recommend that the cardiac patient start at a heart rate of 60% to 70% of the heart rate safely achieved during exercise treadmill testing. This intensity is then gradually increased to 75% of the individual's maximum heart rate as the patient progresses. Increases in effort are made according to the patient's motivation and physical progress.

Patients should be taught how to check their heart rates using the radial artery. In many cases, the Borg scale of perceived exertion can be used to assess workload or work tolerance. All patients should receive instruction on how to monitor themselves during exercise. This will enable them to determine their level of exertion during home activities, and to exercise safely after termination of the formal program.

We focus more attention on the duration of safe, low-level exercise rather than pressing for brisk increases in intensity. Brief sessions of high intensity work are not advisable from the standpoints either of safety or of optimal aerobic conditioning. Individualized, gradual lengthening of the exercise period to the optimal range of 30 to 45 minutes of aerobic conditioning is most appropriate. Certainly additional time is required both before and after the aerobic segment for adequate warm-up and cool-down.

We believe that frequency of exercise is the most important component of the exercise prescription. The patient should be encouraged to initiate a lifetime commitment to regular exercise at a minimum frequency of three days per week. A drive to exercise much more frequently or extensively than the optimal often is a signal of stress-related psychological compulsion in other areas of the patient's life. Since such compulsion may adversely affect health, these psychological factors must be concurrently addressed.

The duration of any given cardiac rehabilitation program is variable, depending upon the patient's medical status. A short program may include six sessions each of aerobic exercises and classes on risk factor management, with arrangements for a home exercise program to follow. Other programs may extend to 24 or even 36 sessions, depending upon the medical situation and the progress of the patient. The objectives are to establish the necessary changes in lifestyle that will reduce the cardiac risk factors significantly. If quality of life is overlooked, little is usually accomplished beyond short-term gains.

Periodic checks on the patient's progress are desirable, especially for those on a home program. Another option would be for the patient to enter an outpatient program which has minimal monitoring capability, but always with properly trained personnel and immediate access to defibrillatory and other emergency equipment.

We find that periodic treadmill testing to assess improvements in working capacity enable us to modify the exercise prescription to achieve the desired training effects. We generally recommend follow-up symptom-limited treadmill tests for cardiac patients at 2, 5, and 12 months following cardiac injury, and annually thereafter.

Results

Rehabilitation programs can achieve a significant reduction in risk factors. Although a large number of patients are motivated to stop smoking as the result of a cardiac event, the hard core remaining tend to continue unless they receive additional encouragement and education in how to stop and how to avoid relapse. Many programs, such as the Houston Cardiovascular Rehabilitation Center,[18] report significant reductions in risk factors and increases in exercise tolerance that persist for a year or more. In the follow-up of obese patients in the Houston program, 76% achieved their ideal weight and maintained it one year after entry into the program.

Morbidity and mortality figures vary from program to program, and the more recent figures tend to be more favorable to rehabilitation than earlier ones. However, with regard to quality of life, there is no question that rehabilitation can improve patients' mental state, sense of well being, and facilitate the return to normal activities and work.

An Israeli group[19] achieved marked benefits in post by-pass patients who participated in a comprehensive program that included physical training and control of risk factors. During the first year post by-pass, 58.8% of the trained patients returned to the same job held before the operation and 1.9% stopped working, while among a matched group of untrained patients only 20% continued their former work and 26.6% stopped working. Related to this was the fact that 79% of trained patients were free of exertional angina pain after one year versus 53% of the untrained. Treadmill work capacity, blood pressure and smoking behavior improved more among the trained than the untrained and the improvements were still maintained on retest (4.8 ± 1.9 years). More of the trained group also reported having a good quality of life: 73% in the first year, and 55% on retest, versus 45% and 25% in the untrained group.

In a study comparing the effects of home rehabilitation post-MI versus a six-month exercise-based program[20], about the same percentage of each group returned to work after six months; however, at a five-year follow-up, 56% of the rehab group were still fully employed, but only 47% of the home group were working.

As might be expected, benefits are most evident in those continuing their compliance with the maintenance program on a long-term basis. The Houston Cardiovascular Rehabilitation Center[18] boasts an overall maintenance rate of 76%. They believe their recommendation of the purchase of a home bicycle ergometer is partly responsible as it permits individuals to exercise easily and in comfort, perhaps while watching television or reading.

Return to Work

Because return to work is important for an individual's sense of identity and self-esteem, the occupational assessment should be carefully made. There is a tendency on the part of some physicians to be overconservative, particularly if disability compensation or retirement benefits are available. Very few jobs require a high level of physical work and even heavy physical labor is generally intermittent, of the static or static-dynamic type.[21] Studies by Sheldahl, et al[22] with repetitive lifting have shown that this type of exertion does not stress the heart as much as dynamic exercise and poses no more risk than dynamic exercise at 85% of maximal oxygen consumption.

In evaluating a job, psychological stress is an important consideration as this may pose as much or more of a load on the cardiovascular system as physical exertion, particularly for hot reactors. Standardized tests for hot reacting such as we use in our program (see Chapter 6 on SHAPE) could be important. However, the patient may gain more benefit by learning how to cope with and minimize the job stress than by facing the stress of job loss or job change.

While the energy cost of many tasks can be estimated, the evaluation of the myocardial oxygen requirement must also consider environmental factors such as extremes of temperature or noise. At the Borgess Medical Center[23], the actual work procedure is simulated to determine the physical demands. The staff can then assess the patient's capacity in relation to the activity and focus on improving the cardiovascular function, muscular strength, and psychosocial stressors that are directly related to the work procedure.

Positive influences on return to work are the patients own expectation of returning to work, higher educational level, greater family income, less severe angina, and being employed before surgery or MI[24].

Negative influences on return to work are unemployment before surgery, nonwork income, older age, more severe symptoms, and perception that health is poor.[25] While the majority of patients active in the workforce before a cardiac event return to work, only 20% to 30% of patients under 65 who had not been working before the event reenter the work force.[26] The return to work seems to be influenced more by the patient's own perception of his/her health than by the actual extent of disease or disability. Medications that affect mood may be a factor too. Negative effects of propranolol were identified in one study.[27] Bypass patients are less apt to return to work, especially if they have had an infarction, than are patients who have had only an infarction.

Psychological counseling and physician encouragement can increase the rate of return to work among those who overestimate their disability. Vocational counseling or retraining may provide a less exacting job for those whose previous work was too demanding in some way.

Part of the reason for poor employability outcomes, in our opinion, is a projection phenomenon; that is, "My job did it to me." In addition, the preoccupation with vital technical procedures and problems after bypass is apt to preclude the discussion and management of negative life struggles and related problems. The focus is on "managing the patient's treatment" instead of on helping the patient to rehabilitate him/herself. In our experience, those reluctant to return to work can learn to deal with their jobs with the help of behavioral modification and stress management techniques. The individuals must learn to take responsibility for improving their own health and quality of life. This is an essential part of a truly comprehensive rehabilitation effort. Dealing with all real and perceived conflicts is what rehabilitation is all about. That is why we advocate the integration of surgical, cardiological, psychological, and rehabilitative services.

Team Approach

Cardiac rehabilitation should be considered a part of the team effort in caring for the cardiac patient. The average practicing physician, whether the cardiovascular surgeon, the consulting cardiologist or the primary care physician, does not have the time, equipment, or expertise to develop a comprehensive integrated secondary preventive program for the cardiac patient. In our experience, it works best for the rehabilitative personnel to collaborate with the attending physician in preparing the rehabilitative program. Then during the rehabilitation, they report the continuing progress of the patient to the attending physician. Most important is mutual awareness of any adversities that may occur prior to completion of the course of training and the return of the patient to the personal physician. Mutual trust and respect between the attending and the rehabilitative physician are essential for successful patient service.

If you have answered the question "Why now?" to both your satisfaction and that of your patient, the rehabilitation process stands a high probability of success.

References

1. Oberman A. Rehabilitation of patients with coronary artery disease. In: Braunwald E (ed). Heart Disease: A Textbook of Cardiovascular Medicine, 2nd ed. W. B. Saunders Co, Philadelphia, 1984, pp 1384–1398.
2. Cousins, N. The Healing Heart. W. W. Norton and Co, New York, 1983.
3. Hoffman NY. Change of Heart, the Bypass Experience. Harcourt Brace Jovanovich, New York, 1985.
4. Tesar GE, Hackett TP. Psychiatric management of the hospitalized cardiac patient. J Cardiopul Rehabil 5:219–225, 1985.
5. Knapp D, Blackwell B. Emotional and behavioral problems in cardiac rehabilitation patients. J. Cardiac Rehabil 5:112–123, 1985.
6. Anderson MP. Psychological aspects of cardiovascular disorders and rehabilitation. In: Peterson LH, (ed). Cardiovascular Rehabilitation. Macmillan Publishing Co. New York, 1983, pp 94–117.
7. Sikorski JM. Knowledge, concerns, and questions of wives of convalescent coronary artery bypass graft surgery patients. J. Cardiac Rehabil 5:74–85, 1985.
8. Gilliss CL. Reducing family stress during and after coronary artery bypass surgery. Nurs Clin North Am 19(1):103–112, 1984.
9. Dracup K, Meleis A, Baker K, et al. Family-focused cardiac rehabilitation: a role supplementation program for cardiac patients and spouses. Nurs Clin North Am 19(1):113–124, 1984.
10. Taylor CB, Bandura A, Ewart CK, et al. Exercise testing to enhance wives' confidence in their husbands' cardiac capability soon after clinically uncomplicated acute myocardial infarction. Am J Cardiol 55:635–638, 1985.
11. Dracup K, Guzy PM, Taylor SE, et al. Cardiopulmonary resuscitation (CPR) training. Consequences for family members of high-risk cardiac patients. Arch Intern Med 146:1757–61, 1986.
12. Nemec ED, Mansfield L, Kennedy JW. Heart rate and blood pressure responses during sexual activity in normal males. Am Heart J. 92:274–277, 1976.
13. Garcia-Barreto D, Sin-Chesa C, Rivas-Estany E, et al. Sexual intercourse in patients who have had a myocardial infarction. J Cardiopul Rehabil 6:324–328, 1986.

14. Shine KI. Anxiety in patients with heart disease. Psychosomatics 25(10 suppl):27–31, 1984.
15. Papadopoulos C. Sexual problems of the patient with vascular disease. Med Aspects Human Sexuality Nov:28–29, 1986.
16. Miller NH, Haskell WL, Berra K, et al. Home versus group exercise training for increasing functional capacity after myocardial infarction. Circulation 70:645–649, 1984.
17. Thompson PD. The cardiovascular risks of cardiac rehabilitation. J Cardiopul Rehabil 5:321–324, 1985.
18. Peterson LH. Summary and Conclusions. In: Peterson LH (ed). Cardiovascular Rehabilitation. Macmillan Publishing Co, New York, 1983, pp 301–348.
19. Ben-Ari E, Kellerman JJ, Fisman E, et al. Benefits of long-term physical training in patients after coronary artery bypass grafting—a 58-month follow-up and comparison with a nontrained group. J Cardiopul Rehabil 6:165–170, 1986.
20. Erdman RAM, Duivenvoorden HJ, Verhage F, et al. Predictability of beneficial effects in cardiac rehabilitation: a randomized clinical trial of psychosocial variables. J Cardiopul Rehabil 6:206–213, 1986.
21. Franklin BA. Getting patients back to work after myocardial infarction or coronary artery bypass surgery. The Physician and Sports Med 14(6):183–194, 1986.
22. Sheldahl LM, Wilke NA, Tristani FE, et al. Response to repetitive static-dynamic exercise in patients with coronary artery disease. J Cardiac Rehabil 5:139–145, 1985.
23. Leguizamon EE, Garman JF, Visich D, et al. Borgess Medical Center's Institute for Cardiovascular Health and Rehabilitation. J Cardiopul Rehabil 5:398–401, 1985.
24. Stanton BA, Jenkins D, Denlinger P, et al. Predictors of employment status after cardiac surgery. JAMA 249:907–911, 1983.
25. Oberman A, Wayne JB, Kouchoukos NT, et al. Employment status after coronary artery bypass surgery. Circulation 65(suppl II):II-115–119, 1982.
26. Kinchla J, Weiss T. Psychologic and social outcomes following coronary artery bypass surgery. J Cardiopul Rehabil 5:274–283, 1985.
27. Almeida D, Bradford JM, Wenger NK, et al. Return to work after coronary bypass surgery. Circulation 68(suppl II):II-205–213, 1983.

Chapter 15

Counseling on Sexuality

Robert S. Eliot
Anne Garland

Sexual dysfunction is not uncommon and is often a stressful concern to patients, particularly because they are reluctant to talk about it and do not realize that it can often be helped. Sexual problems may also be symptomatic of disease. Many patients feel inhibited in discussing their sexual problems and need the physician's encouragement and "permission" to overcome their reticence. If the physician does not seem sympathetic or comfortable dealing with this area, patients will not open up.

Health professionals who are not used to taking a sexual history will find that it is less awkward than anticipated when integrated into the normal history-taking. An open-ended question such as "Any problems with sexual function?" may be used. If the patient's condition usually leads to sexual problems, a question such as "Has your illness resulted in any sexual problems or concerns?" is effective.[1]

Gendel and Bonner[2] state that "offhand remarks about sex made by physicians and other health professional constitute a major cause of iatrogenic sexual problems and dysfunction, with other sequelae frequently following. Ignoring the topic altogether . . . may produce the same results. . . . A majority of myocardial infarction patients questioned stated they would have wanted to discuss sexual problems with their physician, but neither they nor the physician raised the issue . . . patients are left feeling anxious, and often angry."

From: Eliot, RS: *Stress and the Heart: Mechanisms, Measurements and Management.* Mount Kisco, NY, Futura Publishing Company, Inc., © 1988.

Typical Complaints

Whether persons are in good or poor health, the complaints are much the same. The men present with erection problems; the women complain of being inorgasmic. Unfortunately, men do not say they have erection problems, they say they are "impotent." That denigrating term means "powerless" and we feel it should never be used. Nobody is completely powerless. Do not use it to describe either yourself or someone else. Impotence has a connotation of futility. Yet for 99 of 100 people with erection difficulties, the problem is transient and temporary and often comes from an identifiable cause. It would not make sense for a patient to endure the pain of a stomach ache for 20 years and not do something about it. By the same token, men with erection problems and women who have problems with lubrication or orgasm should do something about them.

The difficulty is that it is "acceptable" to go to someone for help with a stomach problem but not to go for help with a sexual problem. In our society, we talk about sex a lot but we don't really accept that part of a person's being. Society doesn't accept it, and even professional people don't always accept that in one another. Husbands and wives may not really accept it in one another and avoid discussing sex. You can see the lack of communication in couples who have been married many years but are grossly embarassed to talk about their sex life with another person in the room. They never have discussed these things with each other in private, let alone in front of strangers.

Garland[3] has reported a dramatic example of the communication problem with a couple who came to her for marriage counseling. At the third or fourth session, they were to bring a few specific complaints about one another to be discussed. The wife reluctantly started reading her list which included minor things such as not picking up socks, putting empty milk cartons back in the refrigerator, leaving the garage door open, etc. Finally at the very bottom she added that he blows in her ear and she doesn't like it. She broke down and started to cry as she told how she hated having him blow in her ear during lovemaking. She confessed that she hadn't known how to tell him but she had disliked it from her honeymoon to the present. Her husband who had only wanted to please her was devastated. But of course the problem was hers: she should have made her feelings known long before it became a major irritation. Perhaps some morning she could have said, "John, you are one of the sexiest men I know but blowing in my ear doesn't do it for me. I prefer . . ." Communication is a big problem between couples.

In truly good relationships, both members of the couple really want only to show love for the partner. But sometimes they get into game playing and it does not come out that way. Then the relationship deteriorates.

How Problems Develop

It should be emphasized that sexuality is a natural function. It is an innate capacity that each person is born with and will die with. It does not come on at age thirteen and disappear at menopause or climacteric although many people treat their sexuality as if it did. They don't see it as a birth-to-death process.

Even newborn babies demonstrate sexuality in the delivery room: newborn boy babies will have erections in the first few moments after birth, and girl babies will vaginally lubricate within the first few moments after birth. That is a surprise to most people. It shows, however, that the ability to have an erection and the ability to vaginally lubricate are parallel responses and that obviously since newborn infants have not had time to learn these responses, they are innate capacities. It is not something that is learned at age twelve or thirteen. One would think that as we mature and understand our bodies better, the capacity would be fostered and bring increased pleasure with age. But there are two major problems that sabotage that response.

The first is negative conditioning. Someone tells us it is a no-no; it is not right to do it or talk about it; nice girls don't, etc. The other source of sabotage is conscious control: the individual's own thinking and attitude. We may not have much control over the negative conditioning we are exposed to, but at some point we are mature enough to evaluate it and try to see things from a more rational perspective. Negative conditioning, therefore, is something that can be reversed. Conscious control is different. The effect of conscious control is not always perceived because it happens automatically, but it may create problems.

Since sexuality is a natural body function, the ability to respond sexually is similar to other functions necessary for life: breathing, need to sleep, need to eat, need to defecate and urinate, etc. Consider how much body control you have over these other functions. With breathing, if someone says "I want you to breathe 16 times per minute when I say 'Start,' " you may or may not succeed. However, if someone checked you without your being aware and found you had breathed exactly 16 times per minute, you would be pleasantly surprised. If you don't put pressure on the body function, it works just fine. This is even more evident with sleep. If you know you have little time for sleep because you have to get up early, and say to yourself I have *got* to get to sleep, you are apt to toss and turn all night. However, if you had mixed up on the schedule and thought you could sleep late the next day, you would probably sleep like a baby.

Just as worry can sabotage the need for sleep, it can also sabotage sexual responsivity. If anxiety, stress, or tension is put on a natural body function, soon it doesn't work. Garland calls it "spectatoring" or the "four in the bedroom" syndrome. That is, there are two people in the bed and their counterparts are standing in the corner watching and evaluating what they are doing. For many people this is a day-to-day component of their sexual relationship. They are there physically with the partner, but another part of their personality is observing them and rating them and telling them what they are doing right and what they are doing wrong. That is one of the things that is most detrimental to a relationship.

A sexual relationship is not a goal-oriented activity. It is a way of expressing one's feelings and caring for another person. It is individual and personal.

How one chooses to express sexuality is a totally individual decision. It is not a choice made by somebody else. One of the things that is important to get across to patients is the idea that each person is responsible for his/her own sexuality. Women find that harder to understand than men. There isn't a man on earth who can make a woman become orgasmic. There isn't a thing he can do to give her an orgasm. She gives that to herself. She allows that part of her sexual feeling and sexual expression to be shared with him. It comes as a shock to women that they have nobody to blame for their problem. To men, it is like having a concrete block lifted off their shoulders. For years, they believed that if everything went well and both were happy, the man did it; and conversely if things didn't go well, the man did it. But a woman should not be just a passive participant. A relationship is a give and take and it takes two people: both must be equally interested, and both are equally needful.

Sensual vs Sexual

People don't know the difference between being sexual and being sensual. Being sexual is plumbing—penis and vagina. Being sensual is like the electricity—the feeling. A relationship needs both. In an intimate personal relationship, what makes the crucial difference is how you feel about that person and how you believe that person feels about you. By middle age, a person is not apt to have a sexual relationship with someone he/she doesn't really care about. Of course it is physically possible, but the caring, feeling part that makes it all worthwhile is something that comes from the individual personalities and grows through the shared experiences of life. There is no comparison when a relationship has both sensual and sexual elements.

What is really important in a relationship are the feelings that are expressed. When the feelings, the sensuality, the caring, and the chemistry are there, and the tried-and-true day-to-day basis of the relationship has been established, then the sexuality part and the plumbing part usually work.

In a good relationship, the touching, feeling, closeness, and caring are a 24-hour a day activity, not one that starts at 10 PM. If the feeling and caring are only expressed at the eleventh hour, the relationship is probably not the greatest, and the plumbing may not work too well either.

Sexuality In Wellness and Illness

There are many parallels and some differences between sexuality in health and in sickness. If you were to ask the average person with no health problems, "How is your sex life?" Chances are he or she would have some negative input, saying "Unh," or "I don't have any," or report some problems. Similarly, most patients with kidney or lung disease will admit to problems. It seems to be rare to get an initial positive response from the average person, well or ill. Therefore, you can tell patients they are not alone in this—people who call themselves healthy, have the same disillusionment, the same feeling of inadequacy.

The difference is that once you label a person with a diagnosis that person feels that because he has a disease he is not sexual. "I have lung disease, so I'm not sexual." "I'm an amputee, so I'm not sexual." "I have diabetes, so I'm not sexual." Of course, the fact is that if you limit sexuality to those with a perfect medical track record who have never had anything wrong with them, you are disenfranchising perhaps 90% of the population.

Those with medical problems should not be disenfranchised. However, they may need to make some adaptations according to the type of illness. An amputee, for instance, may find some positions awkward. A diabetic perhaps will need to consider the timing of medications. A person with a pulmonary problem or cardiac failure may need extra pillows to aid breathing. An arthritic may be more comfortable with a waterbed. Illness or disability does not mean one is out of the game, only that a new game plan is needed to fit the situation. The important message to give to patients is: "Go to Plan B; don't throw in the towel."

Patients are very receptive to this message. Most of them have lived long enough to appreciate life's values. They want value, enrichment, and quality. So, in both wellness and illness there are snags, but in neither case are they insurmountable.

Complaints of patients with health problems are the same as those of healthy people, but adding a health crisis to the average relationship increases tension. A cardiac patient may first ask "Am I going to live?" The next question is "How am I going to live with worrying about whether or not I'm going to live?" For some, living with the fear of dying seems worse than dying. Stress and anxiety are now being put on top of a natural body function, and that leads to problems.

Rehabilitation

Cardiac patients and others with serious illness go through a period of depression. As has been mentioned, for some patients this may last 3 to 6 months. But by that time they should be pulling themselves out of it. Patients should first be reassured that depression is normal and then be helped to get on with their lives after they get over the depression.

The greatest benefits of cardiac rehabilitation programs are increases in the sense of well being, increases in physical capacity, and greater hope for the future. By the third or fourth session of a rehabilitation program there is a dramatic change in the patients as they begin to realize that they are capable of doing much more than they had imagined they would be able to do. They can also be reassured that the activities in the rehab program probably require energy far above the level needed for sexual activity.

The energy needed for sex is not as great as cardiac patients may believe. The average exertion is no more than 3.7 METS, with a maximum of about 5 METS for less than 30 seconds.[4] Patients recovering from an uncomplicated MI have a pretty good activity tolerance on discharge from the hospital. When the patient can climb two flights of stairs at a moderate rate without complications or breathlessness or go 2 mph on the treadmill at a 10% grade, they are exercising at the rate of 5

METS[5] and should have no problems from intercourse. Of course if a person is into hanging from the chandelier, his heart rate and blood pressure may be higher, but very few go in for that.

Various factors can affect sexual functioning in illness. Cardiac patients, for instance, may have changes in body chemistry because of medications and diet alterations; there may also be changes in lifestyle. They wonder how their partner at home will adjust to all this. Are they going to talk about it? Can they talk about it? Such conversation was stressful back when they were both healthy, but how is it going to be easier with one or both in poor health?

While some medications can change sexual responsivity, a lot of it is subjective. It is difficult to separate effects that may be due to medication and those due to emotional state. You have to treat them as a conjoint question. In many cases, the medications may be used only temporarily or those chosen may have minimal side effects. Changes in dosage or substituting another drug may reduce the problem. These are things physicians need to discuss with the patients. Medications can also alleviate certain problems. For instance, anginal pain and palpitations may be reduced by the use of beta blockade or sublingual nitrates prior to intercourse.

It is advisable for each patient to consider how the sexual relationship is going to continue and what kind of adjustments will need to be made. Without planning, the patient may find everything else taking priority while precious time goes by. Sometimes a little wine can grease the wheels for those apprehensive or shy, but of course too much alcohol may only lead to new problems including decreased performance.

Patients need information and reassurance from their physicians; then each person can talk to his/her partner about how they feel and what they would like to do and see what kind of new ideas they might generate between them. Illness need not be seen as a detriment; it can serve as a catalyst for change, an opportunity and a reason to make alterations.

Some patients may find that by being forced to change their approach their illness can turn out to be the best thing for their sexual relationship. The reason is that couples may go for years and years without ever talking about their personal relationship. And they would have avoided it forever if one had not got sick. Now with one ill, they have to deal with it, and the open discussion can be the catalyst for revitalization. Being bypassed or having a heart attack can thus become the turning point because it makes the individual reevaluate and reassess a lot of things in life, especially the importance of the personal relationship. For some patients, the knowledge that their loved one is staying by them, and is there when they come out of surgery or the CCU is what enables them to go on. So a relationship that may have been taken for granted may take on a whole new perspective and increased importance. As an example of creativity inspired by illness, Garland reports the story of the wife who complained that her husband would not undress in front of her after his bypass operation because he was self-conscious about his scar. They had apparently had a much freer relationship in the past, and she now felt that he was pulling away from her and avoiding intercourse and intimacy. She could not seem to convince him that his scar was acceptable to her. When therapy did not seem to be helping, Garland finally suggested that the wife try the "nightie seduction scene." The wife was quite skeptical as to her husband's reaction, because she had never done that. It took her three weeks to muster the courage to try it; then she reported enthusiastically that it had worked like a charm.

It is unfortunate that wives don't often show their men how much they are wanted. Usually it is the husband courting the wife. Women know the nice feeling of having a man who is special to them show he wants them. Men too enjoy the feeling that a woman special to them really wants them. With this couple, the man needed his wife to show him that he was still attractive to her. Although this approach might seem obvious to others, someone else had to point it out to this woman, and even then it was not easy for her to initiate it.

Thus neither illness nor aging need be seen as endings but rather can open doors to greater creativity. People are more responsive as they age—so older can mean better.

Myths

A lot of us go through our lives fostering myths about our sexuality. They are testimony to our humanness. We are all human and all have needs. It is interesting that as women are taking on many roles and becoming more assertive sexually, men are voicing more complaints. Women no longer are passive recipients of sexual attention, but have their own ideas of what they want, and the men feel threatened. All of a sudden it is the man getting the headache.

This is partly due to the myth that a "real man" is always ready. A man is no more an automatic responder than a woman is. It is ridiculous to assume that if the stimulus is there the man responds regardless of how he feels about that particular person.

Another myth is that sex is acceptable only for those who are young and healthy—that it seems foolish in those who are old or have gray hair. For a lot of people, the youthful perfection of the *Playboy* centerfold is the sexual goal or is even considered the norm. Of course, ordinary, imperfect women are the norm. And in fact older women are sexual, more sexual probably than the very young women in the photographs who have not lived long enough to be really sexual. Actually, Benjamin Franklin noted this.

The ability to feel and to care develops and mellows with time. At a certain point in life, a person tends to reevaluate what life is all about. With it comes the realization that the people that are important aren't by any means gorgeous, they are *real*. They care, they are involved, they respond and have other important qualities.

Most people have difficulty picturing their own parents as sexual. We too may feel that being sexual is foolish when we have several children or have gray hair. But sex is a birth-to-death process. The only person who is not sexual is somebody in the morgue.

Another mistaken belief is that the act must be spontaneous if it is to be good. However, people have times when they feel good and times when they don't. They are not very likely to find an activity pleasurable when they are hurting. Pain and sexual response just don't go together. Patients should work times of intimacy around the times when they feel best. To a lot of people that sounds like planning and seems devious or even "kinky." But for busy people or those with limitations, the truth is that if they don't plan for it, and don't set a time aside for it, chances are it won't take place. It makes sense for a patient who tends to feel worse at 10 PM and better at 9 AM, to try to be with his/her partner at 9 AM instead of 10 PM. There is nothing wrong with planning. In fact, it can be one of the greatest and nicest aphrodisiacs. For instance, if you knew that you were going to spend the weekend with someone that you found especially exciting and sexually stimulating, you would think frequently of the coming liaison between now and then and would find it very pleasurable. Setting a time to be with someone special can be a very stimulating thing, adds the spice of anticipation, and probably helps make the time together go very well.

It is important to assure patients that there is no set goal in a sexual relationship. The only goal is for partners to communicate how each feels about the other, whether or not physical intercourse is part of that expression. The important thing is the closeness, tenderness, and the expressing of affection. Many husbands and wives do not understand this. They assume that if there is no physical intercourse, or if one is inorgasmic, it has been a total waste. Nothing could be farther from the truth. No one can fail in a sexual relationship if they express caring and affection. It is immaterial whether or not there is an erection or an orgasm. The criterion is whether each partner expresses and conveys to the other true feelings of affection.

Another myth is that only the "Missionary" position is normal and acceptable. There is no abnormal position. Normal is whatever is acceptable to the two people involved. In Asian cultures there are over 300 documented, diagrammed positions for intercourse. In Western culture, there are perhaps 2 or 3 commonly used.

For a male cardiac patient it may be much more comfortable to have the partner on top. For a lot of people this requires a major adaptation. For many it is a joyful adaptation, adding spice to a relationship. For others the change is extremely difficult. However, sometimes changing the position can be effective in helping nonorgasmic women become orgasmic. More women are orgasmic when they are on top than when on the bottom, simply because of the anatomy.

Another myth is the one that too much sexual activity causes burnout. One of Garland's patients tried to space out his activity because he heard that one gets only so many orgasms in a lifetime. Since his parents had lived to be ninety, he was trying to limit himself to one a month so they would last for his expected lifetime to eighty or ninety. His wife brought him for therapy because she wanted more.

Providing basic information to such people can eliminate a lot of problems. There are some helpful books such as the following:

Male Sexuality by Bernie Zilbergeld (Bantam 1978), which gives the best insight into what it is like to be a male. Males will find out that they are like everybody else, and females will learn how to better care for the men in their lives.

Love and Sex after Sixty by Robert N. Butler and Myrna I. Lewis (Harper Row 1977), is best read before one is sixty. It shows what the advantages are of aging, and it is well written.

For Yourself by Lonnie Barback (Doubleday 1975, or New American Library for paperback) describes female physiology and what it is like to be female.

References

1. Ende J. Screening for sexual dysfunction. Med Aspects Human Sexuality 20:10–14, 1986.
2. Gendel ES, Bonner EJ. Sex, angina, and heart disease. Med Aspects Human Sexuality 20:18–36, 1986.
3. Garland A. Personal communication.
4. Green AW. Sexual activity and the postmyocardial infarction patient. Am Heart J 89:246–252, 1975.
5. American College of Sports Medicine. Guidelines for Graded Exercise Testing and Exercise Prescription, second edition. Lea & Febiger, Philadelphia, 1980, p 19.

Chapter 16

Achieving Compliance (Adherence)

Robert S. Eliot

Introduction

The key to effective treatment, whether therapeutic or preventive, lies in adherence to recommendations. Without the cooperation of the patient no medication or behavioral plan can work. And the key to good compliance lies in the physician-patient relationship.

Some of the reasons given for poor compliance are the following[1]:

a. The patient did not understand the physician's directions.
b. The patient did not wish to relinquish control of his care to the physician.
c. The patient was not convinced of the need or efficacy of the treatment.
d. The patient did not think the treatment was very important.
e. The treatment was too expensive.
f. The treatment was too inconvenient.
g. The patient forgot.
h. The treatment made the patient feel worse.
i. The patient felt all right and decided further treatment was not needed.
j. The patient thought the doctor did not understand him or his problem.

From: Eliot, RS: *Stress and the Heart: Mechanisms, Measurements and Management.* Mount Kisco, NY, Futura Publishing Company, Inc., © 1988

Good communication between patient and physician can obviate most of these conditions. This requires that the physician himself or one of his staff take the time to explain the reasons for the proposed treatment, the health consequences of neglecting treatment, and the proper methods for carrying out the therapy. It is desirable to have the patient repeat the directions in his/her own words to verify that they are understood. I find that recording directions on audiocassette is a great adjunct, because patients often cannot remember instructions given once only. This also permits the spouse or other supportive person to learn the details.

Some patients may gain an advantage from the sick role. Advantages may be financial support, freedom from unwanted responsibility, or increased attention from the family or physician. It is almost impossible to gain compliance if the patient does not want to improve his health.

Depression that often accompanies cardiovascular ailments may blur perception and make the patient feel that treatment is a waste of time—that his condition is hopeless. Reassurance and treatment for the depression must then take priority over other rehabilitative measures.

Rapport between the physician and patient is necessary for gaining compliance. The physician must understand the concerns of the patient with regard to maintaining control, financial or marital problems, overmedication, etc. A patient who feels the physician is too authoritative may ignore the physician's advice or set his own timetable and thereby gain a false sense of control. A patient who has been treated perfunctorily and given a prescription off-handedly, may assume that neither the illness nor the treatment are of much importance. It is then very easy to "forget" to take medication, to neglect refills when money is short, or to decide not to bother because it probably wouldn't make any difference anyhow.

On the other hand, a high rate of compliance can be achieved if the therapy team has tailored the plan to the patient's lifestyle, explained the plan, the rationale, and the importance of the treatment, showed that they *care* about the patient's health, and reinforced this with regularly scheduled follow-up visits, phone reminders, or checkups. Support groups of patients with similar disorders also can be of help, as they have common concerns. By sharing experiences, they can learn useful coping strategies as well as psychological support.

Compliance has been found to correlate with the explicitness of the physician's instructions, and instructions tend to be more explicit the more questions the patient asks.[2] However, few patients ask questions, even when they do not understand. Garrity,[2] describing a study by

Svarstad of 131 low-income patients and 8 physicians at an urban health center, writes, "female patients, Spanish-speaking patients and patients with presumed past experience with the medication received less explicit instruction. Neither patient's age, education, nor the number of patients in the clinic awaiting attention appeared to influence explicitness of the physician's instruction."

Frequent contact with health professionals and/or encouragement from spouse and family increases adherence to the prescribed regimen. Written contracts spelling out what the patient is to accomplish and signed by both patient and physician have been found effective in many cases, especially if the family is also included.[3] The contract may even specify rewards for successful accomplishment of the terms.

As I mentioned, an audio tape of the physician's suggestions and explanations that can be replayed for verification and reinforcement can help patients maintain the proper treatment. Written instructions, if easily understood, can serve the same purpose.

Various other strategies can make it easier for patients to comply with therapy. Some of these are described below.

Antihypertensive Medication

The major reason for failure in patient compliance is the silent nature of the disease and the "noisy" nature of the therapy. Since many a patient is made "ill" by therapy, appropriate adjustments must be made and adequate communication must exist between patient and physician. A patient can also be uncooperative or noncompliant when, at the subconscious level, he may be trying to say, "Doctor, you are not listening. It's my mother-in-law, not my blood pressure that's bugging me!" Thus, the divergence of concern between a psychosocial problem, which concerns the patient, and the diastolic pressure which concerns the physician, may preclude therapeutic harmony.

Finally, as much maturity, independence, and responsibility as possible must be retained and sustained by the patient. The assumption of a dependent relationship with a physician is one which is regressive and intolerable to some. It is recognized that a fraction of patients welcome the opportunity for total dependence and pill taking. Most patients, however, welcome discussions on the maintenance of independence. This could even lead to formal agreements between physician and patient allowing the patient some active responsibility in the control of his own disease. The physician must discover or create positive motivations for each patient and reinforce them. For example, "How interested are you in controlling your blood pressure?" or "You have an excellent chance of avoiding your father's problem."

The medication schedule should be kept as simple as possible. It has been found that patients have more difficulty with pill-taking the more medications that are prescribed.[4] It is essential for the physician treating hypertension or other cardiovascular ills to be aware of the other medications a patient is taking; this is important because of possible interactions as well as for simplifying the regimen. For example, it has been noted that, on average, the post-bypass patient has more than six prescription medications.

Cuing the time of taking medications to other repeated actions such as brushing teeth or mealtimes has proved to be the best way to maintain compliance in cooperative patients.[5] Another strategy is to place the medication in a place where it is easily remembered.[6] For many busy or elderly people, it is helpful to be reminded by someone else who is more time conscious. Special pillboxes with labeled slots are especially useful for those with a complicated regime; these can be filled once a day (some even cover an entire week) with all the required pills, and a forgetful patient can see at a glance whether he or she has taken the scheduled dose already and when the next medication is due. (For liquid medications, bits of color-coded paper can be inserted as a cue and discarded when the dose has been taken.) Another possibility is a written chart with boxes to be crossed off as each dose is taken.

Disturbing side effects are a frequent reason for discontinuing antihypertensives. If an analysis, such as our SHAPE program, has identified the mechanism by which the blood pressure is raised, and the medication is tailored to the individual's needs, the likelihood of side effects is considerably decreased. In any case, the patient should be reassured that medications can be changed if undesirable side effects do occur. Impotence does not enhance compliance!

Reinforcement and verification of compliance are aided by prescribing just the amount of pills needed until the next regularly scheduled checkup. When the patient comes in, any problems with the medication can be discussed and changes made as necessary. If the patient misses an appointment, obviously he/she is noncompliant and followup is even more urgent.

Diet

Drastic changes in diet are rarely maintained for more than a short time. The key to long-term compliance lies in minimizing the changes or spreading them over the long term, gradually introducing new foods to substitute for familiar, less healthful ones.

Most families have a basic pattern of food menus involving about a dozen recipes. The best way to institute permanent changes in diet is to revise these same recipes to reduce the cholesterol, salt, and sugar. With a dietician's help this is possible for a wide range of recipes.

Another strategy patients can use is to change the size of portions —decreasing the amounts of red meat and rich desserts and increasing the amounts of vegetables, salads and whole-grain products. Also, the number of meals featuring red meats can be cut down, replaced by meals centered on chicken, fish, or vegetable protein.

The physician in charge should consider which aspects of dietary change the patient finds most onerous and try to determine whether that change is really necessary. For instance, the elimination of salt does not significantly affect the blood pressure of some hypertensives. If vegetables seem unappealing without flavoring from butter or salt and none of the various salt substitutes seems palatable, it may be better to permit the salt than to have the patient fill up on meat or to give up on the diet altogether.

Often individuals are unaware of the cues or circumstances which lead to bad food habits. Beware of eating patterns such as morning anorexia and evening binges. A food diary for a few days can reveal patterns that can be altered or improved with slight changes that are acceptable. Pre-dinner snacking could be in the form of dry cereal bits instead of nuts; coffee and doughnut breaks could be Perrier and whole-wheat toast; "special treats" for the family could be exotic fruits instead of boxes of candy.

Exercise

Individuals who have little interest in sports and enjoy a sedentary existence can always find excuses for avoiding exercise—bad weather, a backache, a pressing engagement, a scheduling snafu. . . . The challenge is to incorporate exercise into regular daily activities. Although a close-in parking spot is a coveted perk, it may be possible to convince people that a distant spot requiring a five-minute walk is really better for their health. Taking the stairs instead of the elevator also provides an easy exercise.

The high rate of compliance of the Houston group[7] discussed in the chapter on cardiovascular rehabilitation is attributed to their recommendation for home bicycle exercisers. Their patients need not travel to a gymnasium or endure the heat or cold of the outdoors, and can even watch their favorite TV show while exercising. Of course, calisthenics and other types of exercise can be done at home but perhaps expensive equipment increases one's commitment. At least, it is worth suggesting to those who do not particularly enjoy sports or jogging.

Smoking

Motivating patients to discontinue cigarette smoking can be one of the hardest tasks. A confirmed smoker not only has a chemical addiction but a "coping pattern" and a device to establish social interaction and support. Substitutions must be made for all these aspects of the behavior.

The temporary use of nicotine gum has been found helpful in dealing with the chemical addiction.[8] Practicing relaxation techniques may establish a new coping pattern. But substituting socialization at the water cooler for the smoking room may prove more difficult. For many people, antismoking groups work better than solitary attempts to stop smoking.

It is important to determine what situations are associated with the patient's smoking behavior so that he/she can avoid them as much as possible while establishing the nonsmoking behavior. For instance, if the patient generally smokes at parties it may be advisable to give up such social occasions for several weeks to eliminate the smoking cue. If the patient usually lights up after finishing a meal, he/she may find it helpful to leave the table immediately after eating and start another activity not associated with smoking.

Patients should also be instructed beforehand how to deal with a backsliding incident—not to immediately regard the project as hopeless and take a guilt trip. Instead, they should view it as a minor relapse with each new day presenting new opportunities for success. Keep quitting until it works, since each new attempt carries a success likelihood of 30%.

One obvious stumbling block to change would be the physician who smokes or allows his staff to smoke. The recalcitrant smoker can easily rationalize that if his doctor really believed smoking was so detrimental he wouldn't indulge himself or permit those under his supervision to do so. Fortunately, few physicians continue to smoke, and increasing social pressure through environmental restrictions has removed smoking from the realm of "normal" behavior.

Cognitive Restructuring

Even well-motivated patients find behavior difficult to change unless they are given clear instructions on how to proceed step by step. Reinforcement in the form of person-to-person contact is the most effective method of obtaining compliance.

Strategies cued to other aspects of life may help some patients alter their negative thinking. For instance, a patient might be advised to praise himself for something done well that day as he brushes his teeth each evening; or an appropriate reminder such as "smile," "slow down," or "listen," might be posted in a prominent place. Even inconspicuous cues, such as rubber bands or tiny stick-on dots, can be used as reminders if the patient associates them with the desired behavior.

Compliance is also aided if the individual envisions the needed change as a series of achievable goals and rewards himself/herself as each goal is reached.

References

1. Cummings KM, Kirscht JP, Binder LR. Determinants of drug treatment maintenance among hypertensive persons in inner city Detroit. Public Health Rep 97.99–106, 1982.
2. Garrity, TF. Medical compliance and the clinician-patient relationship: a review. Haynes, RB, Mattson ME, Engebretson TO, (eds). Patient Compliance to Prescribed Antihypertensive Medication Regimens: A Report to the National Heart, Lung and Blood Institute. NIH Publication No, 81-2102, Oct, 1980, pp 113–138.
3. Cialdini RB. Mobilizing patients to be committed to the treatment plan. Physician & Patient 4(2):43–46, 1985.
4. Eraker SA, Kirscht JP, Becker MH. Understanding and improving patient compliance. Ann Intern Med 100:258–268, 1984.
5. Levine DM. Cuing—adapting medication-taking to normal living habits. Physician & Patient, 4, 35–38, 1985.
6. Peck CL, King NJ. Increasing patient compliance with prescriptions. JAMA 248:2874–2877, 1982.
7. Peterson LH. Summary and conclusions. In: Peterson LH, (ed). Cardiovascular Rehabilitation: A Comprehensive Approach. Macmillan Publishing Company, New York, 1983, pp 301–348.
8. Hjalmarson AIM. Effect of nicotine chewing gum in smoking cessation—a randomized, placebo-controlled, double-blind study. JAMA 252:2835–2838, 1984.

Chapter 17

Prevention

Robert S. Eliot

Role of the Physician

Physicians and other health personnel can play an important role in prevention of cardiovascular and other diseases. Patients are much more responsive to recommendations for behavioral change made by their own physicians than to exhortations by the popular press, family, or friends. It has been estimated that each family physician has the opportunity to help twenty-five persons per year to stop smoking; in a decade the impact can be tremendous.

Physicians also have a strong influence on the society in general. Through their own behavior as role models and their advocacy of good health practices in the organizations and groups to which they belong, they can gradually improve the acceptable standards—decreasing the acceptability of cigarette smoking in public, the "necessity" for alcoholic beverages (especially in excess) at social gatherings, the equivalency of rest breaks with breaks for coffee and high-caloric sweets.

Change is Difficult

The most dramatic example of the clinical difficulties involved in changing behavior is the Multiple Risk Factor Intervention Trial (MRFIT).[1] This ten-year trial seemed to provide ideal circumstances for behavior modification. The subjects consisted of people in the top ten

From: Eliot, RS: *Stress and the Heart: Mechanisms, Measurements and Management.* Mount Kisco, NY, Futura Publishing Company, Inc., © 1988.

percent risk category for heart disease who were aware of their risks and were motivated to participate. They volunteered to join in the program with the explicit understanding that they would change their smoking behavior, their diet, and even take pills if necessary. The intervention plan used was a "state-of-the-art" model and was implemented in the twenty-two MRFIT clinics by a superb highly trained staff who worked with these individuals for over six years. It is hard to imagine a better circumstance for producing maximal behavior change, yet smoking behavior was reduced by only 50%, and only 50% of the goal in reducing cholesterol levels was achieved. This study indicates the extremely limited role of one-on-one behavior change.

As Leonard Syme[2] has pointed out, in view of the large and extensive incidence of heart disease in our population, (seven million Americans currently have heart disease) treating present patients on a one-on-one basis would involve 28% of physician time (excluding only specialists such as dermatologists, psychiatrists, anesthesiologists, pathologists, etc., who are not likely to treat this disease). And still individuals would continue to enter the disease population at a rapid rate.

Expanding this model to include the new entries would still not alter the social forces in our environment that promote vulnerability to coronary disease and add over a million to the at-risk group each year. In a nutshell, we would have exhausted medical resources in this country and still remained at square one. Obviously we need a broader view that encompasses the forces in the environment. Although useful on the individual level, overall, behavioral intervention can be expected to have only a modest impact as long as we live in a society that unwittingly sets the stage for these troubles in the first place.

So the first problem is that it is difficult (but not impossible, in our experience) to get people to change on a one-on-one basis. Second, even if we had a perfect intervention scheme, there would still be a large population continually entering the at-risk group. Third, even if we could attack all the well-known risk factors at this time, these account for less than 50% of all new coronary events.

Nevertheless, as we have already stated, the risk factors are significant for prediction. An individual who has a single one of the three major risk factors—high cholesterol, hypertension, or cigarette smoking—has double the population risk. An individual with two of these risk factors has $3\frac{1}{2}$ times the risk, and with all three, the risk is six-fold.[3] Yet in populations that have all these risk factors, the vast majority never get heart disease. Indeed, in the community studies of Marmot and Winkelstein[4] in a ten-year period only 14% of men with all three risk factors got heart disease, and among those that did get heart disease, only 58% had at least two of these risk factors. Thus the problem cannot be dealt with merely on a one-on-one basis.

It is difficult for an individual to change unhealthful habits even when he is aware of their effect on his health and has been advised by his physician. It is virtually impossible to change if the environment provokes the unhealthful behavior and is not supportive of the more beneficial lifestyle. We must face also the need to alter the environment to be supportive to the individual.

Changing the Environment

As Syme[3] has pointed out, buildings could be designed to facilitate the use of stairs by having the stairwells built in the center area and as accessible as the elevators. Architects are concerned primarily with esthetics or economy and rarely design with health in mind. We don't have showers readily available in our workplaces. In the supermarket, the healthful foods are usually on the bottom shelf and are expensively priced whereas the "junk food" is frequently at eye level and attractively priced. Teen-agers report that peer pressure in school makes it easier to smoke than to resist. It is difficult to change behavior alone; it is much easier if the physical and cultural environment is supportive.

The environmental-community approach to behavioral modification has been tried. The campaign in North Karelia, Finland,[5] demonstrates that the prevailing mode of behavior can be changed with beneficial results. Over a period of ten years, the use of educational programs in the schools, publicity in the media, and home visits by public health workers, succeeded in significantly reducing smoking among men and in lowering the mean serum cholesterol level about 12%. Concurrently, the CHD mortality among middle-aged men declined 27%. But during my visit there in September, 1986, I found they still had a long way to go.

In the United States too, the noteworthy reduction in CHD mortality over the past decade can be largely attributed to increased public awareness and changed attitudes to smoking, high cholesterol foods, and exercise. One can now advocate such things as high-fiber food, aerobic exercise, and smoking cessation, without being labeled a "health nut." Unfortunately, most of the benefit is stratified, success being found mainly in the upper socioeconomic levels. Blue-collar workers and lower socioeconomic groups have not yet markedly reduced their cigarette smoking and serum cholesterol levels—and CHD rates.

Kotchen and her group[6] have made a notable contribution in this regard by showing that a community-wide, multifaceted approach to hypertension control could significantly reduce the incidence of and mortality from cardiovascular disease in a rural mining area. The effort included educational programs disseminated through the media, schools, and community organizations; blood pressure screening and monitoring; and special contact with individuals targeted by physicians for aid in reducing cardiovascular risk factors.

Dr. Syme is now trying a community-project approach to smoking cessation in Richmond, California. This environmental approach attempts to foster the discontinuance of smoking by changing the way in which smoking is perceived by the entire community. It will involve working with schools, developing block captains, making movies, enlisting the support of all the physicians in town, and involving as many people in the community as possible. The goal is to put smoking on the agenda of the entire community; to say to the community that smoking is not normal, acceptable behavior. It is most unusual for people to feel that this type of issue merits changing the social climate of a whole community. This approach should certainly help individuals to stop smoking, since they won't be faced with all the provocative factors present in most communities. Development of a supportive environment to aid smoking cessation is an important new step that goes well beyond those attempted in the MRFIT program. If this ambitious five-year project succeeds, it may apply to many societies.

Whether through community-based projects such as Syme's or the one-to-one influence of health practitioner and patient, the most important focus of prevention is children. Smoking, overeating, and sedentary lifestyle are hard to change once they have become established. Good habits developed early in life will endure and even carry over to following generations. However, individuals can change at any age and obtain some benefit.

Drawbacks

Efforts to change overall lifestyles necessarily impact persons not actually at risk, and may even endanger a few people: lowering cholesterol levels seemed to increase the mortality from noncardiovascular causes; too great an emphasis on avoiding obesity may increase the incidence of anorexia; treatment of mild hypertension causes distressing side effects in many people which counterbalances the benefits to a large degree. The Pooling Project Research Group[7] estimated that even among those healthy male adults 40 to 55 years old at highest risk according to their cholesterol levels and blood pressure two thirds would remain fit over the next 25 years.

Targeting Those at Risk

It would seem prudent to identify those at greatest risk and concentrate greater efforts on these few. Prime candidates, then, would be close relatives (parents, children, and siblings) of patients who have developed evidence of CHD before 50 years of age. The American Heart Association recommends that such family members be screened for serum cholesterol and blood pressure levels. Stress testing, I think, would also be advisable.

Hot reactors, determined either by a routine screening procedure or tested because of particular problems, are among those at particular risk, in my opinion.

Evaluations of the accepted cardiovascular risk factors are useful in identifying the 10% of the population who will suffer almost half the cardiovascular-related morbidity and mortality. Among these, the elderly constitute an obvious high-risk group, but persons in high-stress situations or occupations, such as transit workers, media reporters and producers, city editors, lab technicians, air-traffic controllers, firemen, police officers, and especially single parents, would seem deserving of special attention.

To prioritize prevention, one can concentrate on the population at risk by utilizing equations based on the results of the Framingham Study.[8] With these, it is possible to develop a composite score or cardiovascular risk profile for individuals. Handbooks available from the American Heart Association and the National Heart, Lung and Blood Institute contain a formulation employing the risk factors of serum cholesterol level, systolic blood pressure, glucose tolerance, presence of left ventricular hypertrophy, and cigarette smoking. Thus a good history (including smoking habits and family history) and a few tests for blood pressure, serum cholesterol, blood sugar, etc. can identify the 10% of the population among whom 22% of coronary heart disease, 31% of occlusive peripheral arterial disease, 43% of cerebral infarction, and 40% of congestive heart failure will occur. Among the elderly, it pinpoints the one tenth of that age group among whom half of the strokes and a third of coronary events will occur.[9] Obviously, postponing or preventing strokes tends to prolong a good quality of life at any age, although vigorous preventive measures are not reasonable where advanced pathology is already present or where the treatment has adverse effects on the individual.

Diabetics and hypertensives are among those at especial risk for cardiovascular disease. Physicians treating them for their primary disease may become aware of other prognostic signs. Measures to reduce additional risk factors may prevent or delay more serious developments.

Risk Factor Reduction

Cigarette Smoking

There is little controversy over the health benefits of reducing the extent and amount of cigarette smoking. Good studies show that the most powerful factor in arresting atherosclerosis is smoking cessation. For adults this is very important (although nonsmokers seem to be out of luck). The problem is compliance. Women on oral contraceptives especially should be made aware of the increased risks of smoking, such as a tenfold greater risk of heart attack than nonsmoking users of these contraceptives.

Hypertension

Treatment of moderate and severe hypertension has been shown to reduce strokes and improve survival. Indeed, the effective treatment of hypertension is frequently credited for the remarkable decline in cardiovascular mortality, particularly from strokes, that has occurred in the past decade. The Veterans Administration Cooperative Study[10] and other large scale studies have demonstrated that the benefits correlate with the degree of blood-pressure control. Even among those with mild hypertension (90 to 104 mmHg) mortality is significantly reduced when the blood pressure has been kept under control. In one such study, the Hypertension Detection and Follow-up Program,[11] five-year mortality among mild hypertensives aggressively treated was reduced 20% with a 45% reduction in stroke and a 46% reduction in MI as compared with the "referred care" group.

Sedentary Lifestyle

Much research supports the relationship between health and activity level. Paffenbarger's study of Harvard alumni[12] correlated survival and calories expended at every activity level. Differences have been reported for those expending 500 calories per week, or 20 minutes of activity per day as compared with similar individuals of sedentary habits. While men have been the subjects of almost all studies with regard to CHD and cardiovascular diseases, women also benefit from exercise by its retardation of osteoporosis. Whether there is added benefit from vigorous exercise is controversial; certainly, added hours of exercise and strenuous exertions increase the likelihood of orthopedic injury. Levels of exercise that bring the heart rate to 75% of estimated maximum for thirty minutes three times per week have proved sufficient for cardiovascular benefit. We do not advocate more vigorous workouts or the expenditure of more than 3500 calories per week.

Alcoholism and Drug Abuse

Excessive drinking, by its effects on potassium loss and on cardiomyopathy, is one of the risk factors in sudden cardiac death. It may also raise blood pressure approximately 1 mmHg for each daily alcoholic drink. Of course, alcoholism and drug abuse are associated with other dangerous consequences. With professional help, improved methods of stress management and the development of alternative sources of social interaction can replace these behavioral crutches.

Obesity

Where diabetes, glucose intolerance, or hypertension are also present, benefits can be expected from weight reduction, even if ideal weights are not achieved. The main goal should be elimination of concomitant risk factors.

Cholesterol

Although high serum cholesterol levels (above 240 mg/dL) should signal diet modification in those otherwise at high risk for CHD, the reduction may not be beneficial to others. Clearly this is an area to be determined on an individual basis. However, there is no doubt that improving nutrition is desirable. The Mediterranean type of diet is a reasonable recommendation for reducing cholesterol as well as improving nutrition in general and is probably safe for most normal individuals. This cuisine emphasizes complex carbohydrates such as noodles and rice; vitamin-rich vegetables and fruits; fish and chicken rather than red meats; and olive oil, a monounsaturated lipid.

Social Support

The need for increased social support is evident in many isolated individuals and in those dealing with chronic diseases, either as a patient or caretaker. Health professionals may aid such people by putting them in touch with others having similar problems. There are many formal organizations in existence: for chemical dependents, alcoholics, families of alcoholics, recently widowed, single parents, parents of retarded children, arthritics, etc. These organizations provide an effective emotional outlet and a support system for people in need and often are also a valuable source of information on such things as useful devices, new developments, and coping strategies. Social service departments of hospitals or government agencies usually have lists of such support groups.

Stress Management

As we have emphasized throughout this book, stress management is important in the prevention of disease in general and cardiovascular diseases in particular. For many patients the physician can play an important role by helping them to identify and cope with the stresses in their lives. Motivated individuals may be able to achieve significant improvement on the basis of physician guidance and a good source book. My patients tell me that my book *Is It Worth Dying For?*[13] and the self-teaching audio- and video-cassettes I have prepared have been quite helpful to them.

For those requiring more intensive behavioral treatment, referral to a qualified psychologist may be indicated. Cognitive and experiential therapy such as is practiced at our Institute usually requires no more than a few months, and need not represent a long-term expensive treatment. Group sessions on stress management are effective and are acceptable to most people, even those who are put off by implications of any sort of "mental" therapy. The results can enhance physiological, metabolic, and endocrine changes as well.

Future Trends

Present trends in lifestyle improvement and advancing medical treatment portend continuing reductions in cardiovascular disease. The rate could be increased, however, if prevention were given a higher priority by the health professionals. Fletcher[14] reported on the lack of training in this area among programs for residents, noting that the percentage of patients in teaching hospitals receiving even vaccinations or other simple preventive services is low.

References

1. Multiple Risk Factor Intervention Trial Research Group. Multiple Risk Factor Intervention Trial: Risk factor changes and mortality results. JAMA 248:1465–1477, 1982.
2. Syme SL. Socioenvironmental factors in heart disease. In: Beamish RE, Singal PK, Dhalla NS, (eds). Stress and Heart Disease, Martinus Nijhoff Publishing, Boston, 1985, pp 60–70.
3. Syme SL. Sociocultural factors and disease etiology. In: Gentry WD, (ed). Handbook of Behavioral Medicine, The Guilford Press, New York, 1984, pp 13–37.
4. Marmot M, Winkelstein W Jr. Epidemiologic observations on intervention trials for prevention of coronary heart disease. Am J Epidemiol 101:177–181, 1975.
5. Puska P, Salonen J, Nissinen A, et al. The North Karelia project. Prev Med 12:191–195, 1983.
6. Kotchen JM, McKean HE, Jackson-Thayer S, et al. Impact of a rural high blood pressure control program on hypertension control and cardiovascular disease mortality. JAMA 255:2177–2182, 1986.
7. Pooling Project Research Group. Relationship of blood pressure, serum cholesterol, smoking habit, relative weight, and ECG abnormality to incidence of major coronary events: Final report of the Pooling Project. J Chronic Dis 31:201–306, 1978.
8. Kannel WB, Stokes J III. The epidemiology of coronary artery disease. In: Cohn PF (ed), Diagnosis and Therapy of Coronary Artery Disease. Martinus Nijhoff Publishing, 1985, pp 63–88.
9. McGee DL. The probability of developing certain cardiovascular diseases in eight years at specified values of some characteristics. In: The Framingham

Study. Section 28. U.S. Department of Health, Education and Welfare, DHEW Publ No (NIH) 74-618, Washington D.C., 1973.

10. Veterans Administration Cooperative Study Group on Antihypertensive Agents. Effects of treatment on morbidity in hypertension. II. Results in patients with diastolic blood pressure averaging 90 through 114 mmHg. JAMA 213:1143–1152, 1970.

11. Hypertension Detection and Follow-up Program Cooperative Group. Five-year findings of the Hypertension Detection and Follow-up Program. I. Reduction in mortality of persons with high blood pressure, including mild hypertension. JAMA 242:2562–2571, 1979.

12. Paffenbarger RS, Hyde RT, Wing AL, et al. Physical activity, all-cause mortality, and longevity of college alumni. New Engl J Med 314:605–613, 1986.

13. Eliot RS, Breo DL. Is It Worth Dying For? Bantam, New York, 1984.

14. Fletcher SW. The periodic health examination and internal medicine: 1984. Ann Intern Med. 101:866–868, 1984.

Special Problems

Chapter 18

Eating Disorders: Anorexia, Obestiy, and Dieting

Robert S. Eliot
C. Wayne Callaway

Eating disorders of obesity and anorexia are associated with a combination of inherited tendencies, cultural pressures, and psychosocial stressors. Part of the problem is the confusion of a cultural norm with a health optimum. Our concepts of the ideal body shape and of obesity are culturally defined. Television "role models" are uniformly slim—a powerful nonverbal directive. However, anthropologists are pointing out that in many societies what we call obesity is not only considered healthy but desirable. In fact, researchers in Tucson, Arizona, had to come up with a new Spanish word for fat (*gordamal*) because *gorda* and *gorda-vita* were terms of approval. Yiddish also has a favorable term for plump (*zoftig*). Indeed, almost every language has a term generally implying something nice about a person who is plump. In Germany, obesity in males has been, and still may be, a symbol of affluence and success.

In the United States, which leads the world in its cultural emphasis on slim bodily contours, a large percentage of the population, particularly women, are constantly trying to use low-calorie diets, or even more drastic measures to control their weight. These behaviors have definite health consequences. Thus, another problem in obesity studies is the failure to distinguish between overweight chronic dieters and other "fatties."

From: Eliot, RS: *Stress and the Heart: Mechanisms, Measurements and Management.* Mount Kisco, NY, Futura Publishing Company, Inc., © 1988.

It is of interest that the Seven-Countries study by Keys[1] found no linear relationship between increasing mortality and increasing relative weight. In fact, Keys points out that in several countries the all-causes death rate tended to be inversely related to relative body weight, and that most prospective studies failed to show that overweight was a major risk factor even for coronary heart disease. It is possible, of course, that the higher risk of death in the underweight reflected extant disease. The study also suggests that major risk factors absorb whatever minimal risk is contributed by excess fat under 30% of body weight. Morbid obesity (over 50%) is another matter.

Desirable Weight

The basic question, then, is "what is desirable weight?" Standards, such as those derived from the NHANES surveys, are based on findings for 20- to 29-year-olds and do not allow for age adjustments. According to such standards, by the age of fifty-five, 30% of white women and over 60% of black women would be considered obese.[2] In light of current knowledge, these standards (obesity as 20% above recommended weight for 25-year-olds) are irrational and could easily be considered discriminatory, especially since women live longer than men. Furthermore, the cardiovascular risks related to obesity are significant only in the younger age groups. Over age 45, overweight apparently does not add much to the risk picture.[2]

Andres[3] notes that the body mass indexes (BMI) calculated for the ideal weights of the 1983 Metropolitan Life Insurance Company come to 22.4 kg/m2 for males and 22.5 for females. However, above age 39, these are lower than the BMIs associated with lowest mortality for the various age groups in a study derived from 4.2 million insurance policies. For every decade of life, the average risks of death at the various weights make a U-shaped curve (the extremes of light and heavy weights all have a greater risk than the medians) and the nadir of the U rises with each decade. Andres points out that height/weight tables should be revised upward 10% to 20% for normal healthy persons in the older age groups. Furthermore, the desirable weights for twenty to thirty-year-olds may be slightly too high.

Obesity

The term "obesity" generally means weight at least 20% above the ideal body weight or over 30% total body fat. It is now recognized that there are different types of obesity but most classification systems contain only two divisions: One divides fat types into exogenous or endogenous; another uses belly vs butt; there is also male type vs female; or fat cell number vs fat cell size. But any medical classification system with just two categories is a gross oversimplification. Each category includes multiple subtypes, and some overlaps. At this stage a probabilistic approach may be more helpful than rigid classifications.

A comparison of the two extremes of one of these systems—adult onset abdominal type of fat vs the hip-pelvic adolescent onset type— shows some revealing correlations. The person with the abdominal type is more apt to have large fat cells, cells more resistant to insulin, higher triglycerides (related to the resistance to insulin), diabetes mellitus and hypertension. In the test-tube, belly fat treated with catecholamines releases fat more readily than similarly treated hip fat. That is, the former is more beta responsive, and the latter is more alpha responsive. Fat in the hips is not as easily mobilized with starvation or with adrenaline or norepinephrine. This can be seen in the African women of the Kalahari desert with steatopygia (huge buttocks) who can starve to death with pounds of fat still on board. Apparently the pelvic fat, which often is related to pregnancy and breast feeding, is hormonally determined while the abdominal fat is more calorically determined.

In prospective studies, it has been found that in men a waist/hip ratio above 1.0 is a risk factor for ischemic heart disease, stroke, diabetes mellitus, and death; in women the risks rise with a ratio above 0.8.[4]

Genetic Factors

The recognition of heterogeneity in obesity is necessary for progress in this field. There has been evidence for many years of the genetic element in obesity. (Animal work to breed beasts that gain weight more quickly or produce more butterfat in milk should certainly indicate that.) The hereditary tendency has been convincingly shown in a Danish study of 540 adult adoptees.[5] The body-mass indices of adoptees correlated with those of their biologic parents but not to their adoptive parents.

Of course the genetic elements are not as simple as the single gene for eye color; there are multiple ways to get fat. For instance, in large-scale studies of obese and nonobese persons, no difference can be seen with regard to genetic markers such as HLA (human lymphocyte antigens); but studies of families with some obese and some of normal weight, have shown that the fat members have an increase of certain markers compared to the lean members. Interestingly, a French study describing such a family[6] reported an increase in a different HLA marker from that described in an Italian study. Naturally, if there are different genetic mechanisms, they can be expected to involve different genetic markers. The point is that in large scale studies comparing randomly selected obese and nonobese persons, there would be many variations of HLAs in both groups, and the active markers would be too dilute to have statistical significance.

Obesity and Disease

In the 26-year follow-up of the Framingham heart study, Hubert et al[7] noted a significant relationship between weight at entry and risk of cardiovascular disease. This was more evident in women than in men and could not be attributed to other factors resulting from weight gain. However, the statistics do not show whether any subgroup attempted to normalize their weight, or whether such measures improved or worsened their health. It has been found that the markedly obese, particularly women, are more apt to try drastic diets, and perhaps have a greater risk of cardiovascular damage and sudden death as a result.

In a long-term study of black physicians[8] with regard to CAD and hypertension, it was found that weight on graduation from medical school was not predictive of outcome. Weight after 25 years was a better prognostic indicator, and percent of gain was the best indicator; those who gained a lot of weight in the interim had the poorest prognosis. Obviously, the developmental pattern is important.

Evidently a modest gain in weight with age is not detrimental in the absence of diabetes, hypertension, or other weight-affected disorders. With smoking, the U-shaped curve is similar to that for nonsmokers but indicates higher risk at all weights than for nonsmokers of the same weight (Fig. 1).[9]

We believe it is only necessary to treat categories of obesity that pose an identifiable risk to health. Fitzgerald[10] notes three major categories of risk in obesity: those associated with the increased mechanical burden, the dangers of increased or improper food, and the complications associated with obesity.

Some or all of these risks are certainly present with morbid obesity, defined as 100% above or 100 pounds above average weight. Really, there is not much argument that even 50% above average puts a person at risk for a variety of ailments.

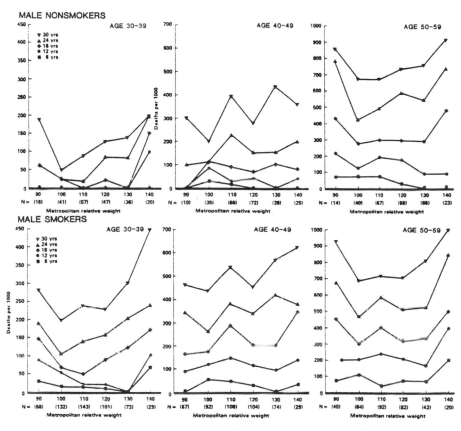

Figure 1: Cumulative deaths per 1000 male nonsmokers (top graphs) and smokers (bottom graphs) according to age group. Reproduced with permission from: Feinlieb, M: Epidemology of Obesity in Relation to Health Hazards, Annals of Internal Medicine 1985; 103(6 pt 2):1019–1024.

We also recommend treatment for those already manifesting a condition such as diabetes, high triglycerides, or high-blood pressure that is known to be benefited by weight reduction. Preventive therapy to avoid obesity is important for those with a strong family history of such conditions. While there is little evidence that weight loss later in life is beneficial, the statistics favor those whose weight is maintained in the desirable range from young adulthood.

Some researchers claim added risk even at 10% above average weight but in my view that is a gross simplification of the data. Some people can maintain themselves very well at a weight that is above our present cultural cosmetic ideal. Perhaps in the future there will be a redefinition of obesity with greater recognition of the heterogeneity and a more precise clinical determination of those at risk, who therefore need to lose weight. Obviously, some people 30% above average are perfectly healthy, especially if they have hip-pelvis distribution rather than predominantly abdominal fat, have been big in the past, and come from families that are generally big. A person like that who may have weighed 220 pounds in the past may come down to 180 and still be overweight, but probably would find it impossible to come down to, say, 140. Fortunately, weight-related problems, such as diabetes and hypertension, often improve with modest weight reduction even though the individual remains above average weight.

Metabolic Rate

There have been studies to try to determine whether fat people metabolize energy more efficiently. Data from the Health and Nutrition Examination Survey I (HANES I)[11] showed that on average skinnier people eat more than fat people. Some physicians may conclude from this that fat people don't tell the truth because the report does not conform to their prejudice.

However, the confusion could result from the heterogeneity of the subjects. Studies rarely define what sort of fat people were included. Fat people who are holding their weight forty or fifty pounds below where they would ordinarily be biologically are already adapted to starvation. Thus they will burn less energy than others who are naturally at that same weight and have never been heavier. If both groups eat the same diet, the reduced-weight persons are more likely to gain because their metabolism is low. The group that is at their biological weight and eating just what maintains them have normal metabolism. On the other hand, people who are fat because they overeat have a higher metabolic rate, since the body's homeostatic mechanisms tend to burn off energy at a higher rate with a greater intake. So depending on what sort of fat persons were studied, data can be found to support almost any hypothesis. A study that gives the metabolic rate just for "fat people" is uninterpretable unless it specifies what kind of "fat people"; i.e., those who have been dieting for fifty years, those who eat frequent large meals exceeding their biological needs, or those who are at a stable weight and have never dieted because they grew up in an environment where fat is beautiful.

Age also makes a difference. In the aged, glucose tolerance declines, partly as a result of resistance to insulin due to increased fat cell size and partly from the lowered production of insulin. Also the number of receptors for norepinephrine declines with aging, so older persons cannot mobilize the fat as well.

Set Points

The idea of there being different metabolically determined "set points" for weight is a useful concept as long as it is not viewed as a rigid "thermostat" that controls in a narrow range. What the set-point observations show is that animals and humans tend to resist perturbations in body weights: that is, with less food the slower their rate of weight loss; and with more food the more energy burned off, slowing the rate of weight gain. The criticism of set point is that it has been characterized in the literature as if it were a straightforward, fixed thing. In reality there is a whole cascade of adaptive mechanisms.

In starvation, for instance, norepinephrine turnover goes down, conversion of thyroid hormone into the active form (triiodothyronine or T3) goes down, and both of these changes tend to lower the metabolic rate so one burns less energy. At the cellular level, the fat cell gets smaller and becomes more responsive to insulin which fosters the storage of fat and glucose and inhibits the release of fat from these cells. On the enzyme level, lipoprotein lipase (the enzyme that gets the fat off the transfer lipoproteins and into the cell) is also sensitive to insulin; with a loss in weight, it too becomes more sensitive, tending to increase the storage of fuel.

Conversely, as a person gains weight, the fat cells get bigger and become more resistant to insulin. It then becomes harder to stuff fat into the cell. Lipoprotein lipase activity goes down; as a result, the triglycerides are not removed as readily from the blood. However, if weight gain in adults expands the fat cells to their maximum capacity, further overeating will initiate the development of new fat cells, with a resulting increase in insulin sensitivity, etc., and weight gain. Unfortunately, subsequent weight loss can shrink the fat cells but does not reduce their number.

Set point thus is really shorthand for a whole series of mechanisms which in the aggregate resist major perturbations of body weight or of energy balance. It does not describe an isolated, well defined entity. It can be moved. For instance, with rapid weight gain in adult life, one can make new fat cells,[12] with new fat cells you have a set point for a greater weight because there is a greater capacity for fat storage. To lower the weight set point, the only methods seem to be vigorous physical activity, cigarette smoking, and amphetamines. Obviously the latter two are not prudent therapeutic measures.

In a study of formerly obese subjects who had maintained their weight for years, Leibel and Hirsch[13] found that these subjects had decreased energy requirements per square meter body surface compared to their requirements when obese and these requirements were below those of any of the normal controls. Despite "normal" body weights, these individuals displayed symptoms associated with fasting: including depression, cold intolerance, and amenorrhea. Those changes suggest that they are below their metabolic set point. The metabolism of such individuals seems to become more normal when they increase their activity level.

People who have lost weight and maintained it at the level considered normal for their height not only have abnormal metabolism, they are abnormal in other ways as well. For example, they may display psychological changes. With starvation, depression scores go up, and perception of time and distance is distorted; also encephalographic changes during sleep indicate that less time is spent in the deeper levels of sleep, and, therefore, the subjects wake up tired even after 8 or 9 hours.[14] Exactly the same thing occurs with the individual whose weight has dropped from an initial level of 300 pounds to 200 pounds and who now has small fat cells. Despite his girth, at that cell size, he is starving. Psychologically he will test out as if he were starving, despite being overweight according to the tables.

Obviously dieting itself is not without risks. Similar problems are seen with very low calorie intake among obese and thin dieters, but drastic consequences are more often associated with the latter.

Anorexia and Bulimia: The High Price of Control and Social Acceptance.

Most anorexic patients are young women. They are generally bright, perfectionistic and have a great need to control their lives. Frequently they are the children of driven parents who are high achievers with lofty standards. These children often feel inadequate and externally controlled. They may also feel that although they cannot perfectly control their lives, they can at least control their bodies; that is, their weight. And in the United States and Western Europe, "perfect" is THIN! Naturally, the need to control may be secondary to other factors such as a bid for attention or the weight requirements for athletics. The average body weights for contenders for Miss America and Miss Finland, for example, have fallen about 8 pounds in the past two decades.

The struggle to be thin may not only involve the use of extremely low-calorie diets, but often includes the misuse of laxatives and self-induced vomiting. Some bulimics alternate binging with purging techniques. Patients may induce vomiting as often as 15 times a day, and there have been reports of patients taking 40 to 60 doses of laxative per day. Even if some bulimics maintain nearly normal weight, their health can be severely compromised.

Evidence of these abuses can be found on physical examination.[15,16] Frequent vomiting causes erosion on the posterior surfaces of the teeth from gastric acids. Finger-initiated gagging may actually cause calluses on the fingers and knuckles, and there may be oral and perioral trauma. Enlargement of the parotid or submandibular glands is often observed. Laxative abuse may be suspected in cases of vague abdominal distress, fecal soiling, and other gastrointestinal disturbances.

Vomiting can cause esophageal and gastric tears. The symptoms and damage resulting from the overuse of laxatives depends on the type of laxative used. The damage can include serious degeneration of the mucosa (cathartic colon) as well as various more easily reversible complaints.

From a cardiovascular standpoint, a very thin person with the basic symptoms—weight loss, binging, purging, amenorrhea—suggests the possibility of cardiovascular complications, particularly myocardial atrophy. When the body lacks adequate nourishment, the myocardium becomes wasted, just like the muscles everywhere else.

The inappropriately small heart portends low cardiac output which leads to such things as low-blood pressure at rest and inadequate blood pressure response during exercise. As was demonstrated in Holocaust studies, the metabolism appears to slow down drastically as a survival response to the equally drastic drop in caloric intake.

Along with low output, there are metabolic problems: hypokalemia and hypomagnesemia occur frequently and the combination sets the stage for constellations of rhythm disturbances.[21,29,30]

Another area for concern is the reduced activity of practically all the endocrines—thyroxin, catecholamine, dopamine, serotonin, etc. The reduction of these elements further impacts the patient's ability to withstand chronic psychosocial and/or physical stress. Low levels of certain hormones and neurotransmitters have been linked to mental illness, such as depression, which is very common in the eating-disordered individual.

By the time changes show up in the electrocardiogram, the damage may already be very serious. Arrhythmias, long QRS durations, conduction disturbances, and prolonged QT intervals are all possibilities.[17,18]

Therapeutic low-calorie diets or supervised starvation designed to counteract morbid obesity leads to the same sort of disorders as anorexia. For example, therapeutic starvation (with supplements of vitamins, potassium, folic acid and allopurinol) of 13 grossly obese patients led to QTc prolongation in seven; episodes of atrial fibrillation in another patient; and torsade de pointes tachycardia on refeeding in one of the seven with QTc prolongation. Weekly ECGs showed no adverse effects before six weeks of starvation, and in general, the more obese tolerated the fast longer than the less obese.[19]

Although liquid-protein diets were designed to avoid the muscle wasting induced by starvation and extremely low-calorie diets, the heart muscle apparently is not sufficiently protected. A number of cardiac deaths have been associated with these diets, and the findings were similar to those seen in starvation and anorexia.[20,21] While timely treatment and careful refeeding has reversed the harmful effects in many cases, the abnormalities sometimes have been found to persist for months afterward.

Myofibrosis, vacuolization of the myocardium, atrophy of the heart, particularly in the left ventricle, and myofibrillar degeneration are typical histological findings in the hearts of those with caloric deficiencies.[22] Thus, one of my main concerns is that psychologists or therapists treating these illnesses without good medical counsel may be unaware or untrained in recognizing the unapparent but profound physiological problems that exist.

In my view, the best approach is the integration of behaviorally oriented practitioners into a team with medical, cardiovascular, and gastroenterologic practitioners. In my experience, it takes this team approach to recognize and deal with the constellation of systemic and affective disorders.

The cardiac status, for instance, may require major therapeutic modifications. Refeeding or reperfusing a metabolically depleted patient with an atrophic heart and a low output may put an inordinate strain on the heart. This can lead to ischemia or even sudden death, as we learned after the liberation of starving prisoners in the Nazi death camps. Some of these concentration camp victims died because of the GIs' good intentions to provide abundant food immediately. The unintentional feeding of the wrong types of food, or too much, too fast, can lead to very serious ramifications for heart function. Heroic, premature refeeding also alters the electrolyte balance, predisposing to sudden death or other serious complications. Cautious, gradual refeeding while cardiac output is monitored noninvasively is critical. Since the immune system also is impaired, noninvasive techniques, such as our system based on electrical impedance output system, are preferred for monitoring to reduce the risk of infection.

While tricyclic antidepressants have sometimes been beneficial in treating anorexics, Gould et al[23] warn that such drugs should be used with care because of their arrhythmogenic potential. Anorexics may have cardiac conduction abnormalities in spite of a normal ECG and/or normal electrolytes.

Psychiatrists report that anorexia is the disease with the highest mortality of any psychosomatic illness—about 6%. That is higher than some forms of cancer!

Rebound Effect

Callaway points out that starvation diets are popular because of the logical fallacy that "I did thus and this followed, therefore one caused the other." Typically, a dieter goes on a diet and loses perhaps thirty pounds (of which fifteen or twenty may be water loss). The person later goes off the diet and gains back thirty-five pounds. As Callaway notes, "The diet gets the credit, and the dieter takes the blame. The diet has really set up the weight gain but dieters don't draw that conclusion."

Not only does the metabolic rate go down on a starvation diet, but adaptation makes it harder and harder to burn off additional weight and easier to gain when the individual goes off the diet. Part of this is because of alterations in appetite. When people who are starving are put into a situation where they have to eat, they tend to overeat. According to psychologists, this is the "restrained eater" phenomenon: if a person has been constantly restraining food intake and then is obligated to eat, it becomes difficult to reimpose control. Sweets and alcohol particularly have been noted to trigger this response. Among biologists studying animals the same behavior is reported although animals are not subject to guilt and haven't heard of Freud! Evidently a biological signal is turned on by eating after a period of deprivation, and sweets and alcohol are prime activators of this appetite response.

Landsberg and Young[24] found in experiments with rats that the sympathetic nervous system was suppressed by fasting and stimulated by overfeeding. This would tend to conserve calories by lowering metabolic rates during starvation and stimulate heat production and calorie expenditure during overfeeding. It might also help to explain the incidence of arrhythmias in refeeding after fasting and in certain obese persons.

How To Help Your Patients

Benefits of Weight Loss

As Kral[25] has pointed out "few studies have documented unequivocal benefits from weight loss per se." It is easier to measure the effects in relation to outcome variables such as blood sugar, triglycerides, and so forth. Losing weight is definitely helpful for Type II diabetes. The diabetic symptoms disappear with weight loss, but recur if the weight is regained. With high triglycerides and with a subgroup of the hypertensives there also seems to be valid evidence of benefit.

The adaptation to starvation causes an acute fall in blood pressure, but this may not persist after weight has stabilized. The drop in catecholamines[31] which causes the fall in blood pressure is part of the adaptation to starvation. However, Stamler et al[26] found that a cohort of men with mild hypertension who stayed in a weight-loss study for 5 to 10 years, did achieve lower blood pressures correlated with loss of weight; they were able to maintain their blood pressures at normal levels even though they did not reach the desired weight levels.

Although it is generally assumed that weight lowering in people who are genetically above average in weight would show benefit, there is no supporting data in the literature proving lower mortality for such people.

Of course, orthopedic problems in weight-bearing areas are undoubtedly improved with weight loss. The knee, for instance, bears the equivalent stress to two or three times the body weight, so even small changes in weight can aggravate or improve problems in this joint by altering the physical stress.[27]

Since changes in appetite and metabolism of the formerly obese favor the regaining of weight it is not surprising that so few people succeed in maintaining the lower weights achieved by dieting. Even dieters using the so-called "prudent diets" rarely maintain their desired weight as long as five years. Nevertheless, as long as drastic and dangerous diets are avoided, weight loss may alleviate some strains on the system, at least temporarily. When combined with exercise, it may also break the vicious circle of increased weight leading to reduced activity that in turn leads to further weight gain.

Stomach stapling is beginning to provide data that confirm that weight loss is beneficial with regard to disease in the morbidly obese. This procedure has a place for those extremely obese who suffer from a life-threatening complication, such as sleep apnea, or very poorly controlled diabetes or hypertension. For these we can show improvements in the risk factors of blood sugar and blood pressure. Mortality data may be long in coming because the criteria for the operation generally require the patient to be under 60 years of age or even younger.

Utility of Basal Metabolism Rate (BMR) Determination

The concept that there is such a thing as an ideal body weight is unfortunate. The desirable weight for an individual can't be found just by pulling out the table. One must consider the weight distribution, when the weight was gained, and whether it was associated with physical or mental complications. Risk factors, family history, developmental history, insulin level, and other pertinent information must be reviewed. If the individual has always had the weight, he/she need not lose as much weight as a person of the same weight who had recently gained fifty pounds. The reason is that someone who has always been heavy probably has more lean body mass—more muscle, more bone, and more fat cells—than a person who had a recent rapid gain. Developmental pattern data can provide clues to causation. For instance, a person who is naturally lean and then suddenly at age 27 joins a commune and gains fifty pounds, probably has a psychological element to the weight gain. In general, a sudden weight change outside the developmental pattern strongly suggests either a psychological or pathological origin.

Resting basal metabolic rates (BMR) can be helpful in several ways. One is that they correlate with eating patterns. In the U.S., about two thirds of overweight women skip breakfast, eat a light lunch and then consume 80% of their calories in the evening. Such women have lower resting metabolic rates than those who eat three or more meals a day. A subgroup of the overweight are overeaters, eating five or six times a day, and they have higher metabolic rates. The test is helpful in confirming the eating patterns reported by the patient.

The second benefit of a BMR is that it gives a specific number, an objective measure of the energy consumption. If people have dieted many, many times, they have usually come to the conclusion that they can't lose weight on 1000 Cal/day, they have to go to 500. If they have been on 500 Cal/day and the physician puts them on 1200 Cal/day, they will gain water back—refeeding edema. They will interpret this in the time sequence: "I went off the diet and I gained weight on 1200 calories, therefore I need to be on 500." However, one can show them that they burn for example, 1450 calories at rest, which may be 15% below the average for a person of that build, but still well above 500 calories. It may seem an enormous amount of food, inconceivable as a weight-loss diet, but the number provides an objective standard for negotiating; it is not a matter of the patient's opinion versus the doctor's opinion. Obviously reeducating the patient is critical to his/her understanding about the adaptation process. Then both can agree on a diet that provides at least basal requirements and the patient can be assured that he/she will lose weight, albeit slowly.

A further benefit of measuring the basal metabolic rate is that it can provide a clue to some other problem. For instance, just recently it has been shown that diabetics who are not well controlled will have higher metabolic rates than predicted, probably because their catecholamine levels are elevated. Those are also the ones who have hypertension. Rarely a case of hypothyroidism will be identified. Occasionally, someone will be in a hypothyroid state with a normal total thyroxin but a high TSH and have an abnormally low metabolic rate or high cholesterol. Some drugs such as lithium might cause this.

Most physicians could get a usable estimate of BMR by calculating 22 Cal/kg. Hospitalized patients on bedrest have been found to burn 22 to 24 Cal per kilogram body weight, on the average.[28] A sedentary person probably burns 20% above that—27 Cal/kg. An individual of 85 kg (187 lb) would be estimated to burn 2100 to 2500 Cal/day and have a BMR of 1870 Cal/day. On 1870 Cal/day, the person then should have a slow sustained weight loss, but might have a temporary weight gain from edema. If the individual's intake has been greatly exceeding the BMR, the new diet should not reduce the caloric level more than 500 Cal/day. As the person stabilizes at the new level, further reductions can be made.

Edema

Too often a woman goes to a physician because of puffiness and the physician says "well women have water retention" and gives her a diuretic without taking a careful history or asking if she has been dieting. Some people who have markedly reduced their salt intake find to their horror that after eating a salty meal, such as a Chinese dinner, they can gain as much as 6 pounds (of water) in a single day. On diuretics the magnitude of the fluctuation can increase from perhaps 5 lb/day to even 10 lb/day.

The time frame for normalization is such that if the intake has changed from an 800 Cal/day diet to a 1700 Cal diet which may be basal, it is possible for the dieter to gain as much as 25 pounds of water during the first two weeks and it may require several months for that to come off. Refeeding edema is probably the most common cause of edema in women in the United States, yet it is neglected and overlooked in edema studies. It is probably a form of kidney adaptation to long-term dieting and starvation (sodium-, potassium-, water-retention).

To treat such people, provide them with at least the calorie level of their BMR distributed into three meals per day, with approximately half their calories as complex carbohydrates. Encourage them to exercise in addition. If they exercise while eating less than that, they do not adapt back to their proper metabolic level, in Callaway's experience.

The time it takes for a person to achieve his/her biological weight on a BMR-based diet will depend on how long and how many times that person has dieted, the degree of fluid retention, and the amount of activity. Patients must be warned that their weight may increase for two or three weeks and then it may level off for several months before there is any weight loss. When they panic, as most do, you need to give them olympic reassurance.

Exercise

A person who exercises in addition to using the BMR-based diet will lose more weight. The amount of exercise need not be extreme. Twenty minutes of aerobic activity three to four times per week is sufficient if they are willing to accept goals that are different from their usual expectations.

The effects of exercise on weight vary from study to study. Variables that should be considered are the severity of the exercise, the degree of overweight in relation to biological set point, and the type of diet the person is on. If the person is eating adequately to meet his/her energy requirements and exercises vigorously (running ten miles per week, for instance), the metabolic rate will stay up for hours after exercise. On the other hand, if a person is on a very low-calorie diet, such as a semi-starvation 800 calorie one, the metabolic rate will be high during the exercise but will drop quickly afterward. Adding exercise to starvation leads to a greater degree of starvation than caloric restriction alone. To prevent adaptive changes in the metabolic rate, therefore, the caloric level should at least equal the caloric requirement at rest.

Since normal day-to-day activities add about 20% to 30% above the resting caloric expenditure, even modest increases in physical activity can lead to a slow and sustained weight loss—without activating complex adaptive phenomena designed to conserve life in conditions of starvation.

For many patients it is better to select normalization of metabolism as a goal rather than reduction in weight. Encourage them to ignore weight and accept the weight at which they level off. As the metabolic rate is brought up to normal they will feel better and have more energy. It also helps them to see progress by showing them the objective evidence that their metabolic rate has risen. Patient rapport and physician support are essential. Although this approach is "new," it has a solid physiologic metabolic basis.

Psychological Factors

Of course, it is true that a few people can go on a diet (a fad diet or any other), lose the desired weight and keep it off forever. These are undoubtedly people who have gained weight as adults with no particular family history of obesity. Probably there are fewer psychological factors involved in causing obesity than is generally believed. Studies demonstrate no psychological differences between individuals who are overfat and those with normal body weight. Psychological abnormalities may exist, however, in the morbidly obese. This, in part, accounts for the bleak track record for psychotherapeutic attempts ranging from "analysis" to behavioral modification in "normal" persons.

However, most persons who attempt weight loss, get metabolically unbalanced and feel guilt and frustration at their failure. The resulting stress may be more harmful than the excess fat. In addition, dieters often suffer the same sorts of emotional disturbances seen in starvation

—depression, irritability, nervousness, etc.[32] Those who have been obese from childhood seem to be more vulnerable to mental problems while dieting than those who gained weight as adults.[33]

Another source of stress is the stigmatization of the obese, particularly obese women. While overt ridicule and prejudice against most minority groups and handicapped individuals are taboo, it is still open season on the obese. Wadden and Stunkard[32] in reviewing the situation report that the prejudice is widespread and includes physicians. The overfat also are discriminated against in the work force. They are less likely to be hired or to be promoted; 18-year-olds who are obese are more likely to remain blue-collar workers than those of more normal weight.

Indeed, a variety of such social prejudices has pulled the obligatory legal chains as well, leading to jurisprudence in exogenous obesity. The National Association to Aid Fat Americans has brought a number of weight-discrimination cases to court.

In one interesting case cited by Callaway, a woman who had been employed as a temporary worker in the post office was denied a permanent position on the basis of her obesity although obviously she was capable of doing the work. Ironically, had she possessed any of the associated risks or complications of obesity, such as diabetes or hypertension, she would have been hired because one can't discriminate against the handicapped in Federal employment.

Although appearance is obviously important from the psychological point of view, the physician needs to know whether the patient is primarily interested in cosmetics or in health. We have to separate the cosmetic from the metabolic.

The goal of a diet should have biological meaning, not be an arbitrary weight standard. Percent body fat is better than weight; fat cell size in abdominal fat would be even better. Insulin levels might be a useful metabolic marker. We need to find a standard that relates to the individual's own physiology.

Most women don't diet for health, but to conform to unrealistic beauty standards. Women's literature is beginning to question the acceptance of a definition of a woman's value based only on externals. Appearance standards make even less sense when racial and ethnic differences are considered. The best help for a "plump" patient may be the assurance that she is okay as she is. All the quack programs in the country are trying to have obesity declared a disease so they can get paid for treating people who are otherwise normal. Each patient deserves to know whether weight loss is recommended for valid health reasons. In each case a proper diagnostic evaluation must precede prognostication and individualized management.

References

1. Keys A. Ten-year mortality in the seven countries study. In: Bostrom H, Ljungstedt N, (eds). Medical Aspects of Mortality Statistics. Skandia International Symposia. Almqvist & Wiksell International, Stockholm, Sweden. 1980, pp 15–36.
2. Van Itallie TB. Health implications of overweight and obesity in the United States. Ann Int Med 103(6 pt 2):983–988, 1985.
3. Andres R, Elahi D, Tobin JD, et al. Impact of age on weight goals. Ann Int Med 103(6 pt 2):1030–1033, 1985.
4. Bjorntorp P. Regional patterns of fat distribution. Ann Int Med 103(6 pt 2):994–995, 1985.
5. Stunkard AJ, Sorensen TIA, Hanis C, et al. An adoption study of human obesity. NEJM 314:193–198, 1986.
6. Apfelbaum M, Fumeron F, Dunica S, et al. Genetic approach of family obesity: study of HLA antigens in 10 families and 86 unrelated obese subjects. Biomedicine 33:98–100, 1980.
7. Hubert HB, Feinleib M, McNamara PM, et al. Obesity as an independent risk factor for cardiovascular disease: a 26-year follow-up of participants in the Framingham heart study. Circulation 67:968–977, 1983.
8. Thomas J, Semenya KA, Neser WB, et al. Risk factors and the incidence of hypertension in black physicians: the Meharry cohort study. Am Heart J 110:637–645, 1985.
9. Feinleib M. Epidemiology of obesity in relation to health hazards. Ann Intern Med 103(6 pt 2):1019–1024, 1985.
10. Fizgerald FT. The problem of obesity. Ann Rev Med 32:221–31, 1981.
11. McCarron DA, Morris CD, Henry HJ, et al. Blood pressure and nutrient intake in the United States. Science 224:1392–1398.
12. Greenwood MRC. Adipose tissue: cellular morphology and development. Ann Intern Med 103(6 pt 2):996–999, 1985.
13. Leibel RL, Hirsch J. Metabolic characterization of obesity. Ann Intern Med 103(6 pt 2):1000–1002, 1985.
14. Grinker J, Hirsch J. Metabolic and behavioral correlates of obesity. Ciba Found Symp. 8:349–69, 1972.
15. Bailey S. Diagnosing bulimia. AFP 29(5):161–164, 1984.
16. Sansone RA. Complications of hazardous weight-loss methods. AFP 30:141–146, 1984.
17. Kalager T, Brubakk O, Bassoe HH. Cardiac performance in patients with anorexia nervosa. Cardiology 63:1–4, 1978.
18. Sandhofer F, Dienstl F, Bolzano K, et al. Severe cardiovascular complication associated with prolonged starvation. Br Med J i:462–463, 1973.

19. Pringle TH, Scobie IN, Murray RG, et al. Prolongation of the QT interval during therapeutic starvation: a substrate for malignant arrhythmias. Int J Obesity 7:253–261, 1983.
20. Van Itallie TB, Yang M. Cardiac dysfunction in obese dieters: a potentially lethal complication of rapid, massive weight loss. Am J Clin Nutr 39:695–702, 1984.
21. Sours HE, Frattali VP, Brand CD, et al. Sudden death associated with very low calorie weight reduction regimens. Am J Clin Nutr 34:453–461, 1981.
22. Alexander CS. Nutritional heart disease. Cardiovas Clin 4(1):221–44, 1972.
23. Gould L, Reddy CVR, Singh BK, et al. Evaluation of cardiac conduction in anorexia nervosa. PACE 3:660–665, 1980.
24. Landsberg L, Young JB. Fasting, feeding and regulation of the sympathetic nervous system. New Engl J Med 298:1295–1301, 1978.
25. Kral JG. Obesity and related health risks. Ann Intern Med 103(6 pt 2):1043–1047, 1985.
26. Stamler J, Farinaro E, Mojonnier LM, et al. Prevention and control of hypertension by nutritional-hygienic means. JAMA 243:1819–1823, 1980.
27. Quinet RJ. Osteoarthritis: Increasing mobility and reducing disability. Geriatrics 41:41, 1986.
28. Calloway DH, Zanni E. Energy requirements and energy expenditure of elderly men. Am J Clin Nutr 33:2088–2092, 1980.
29. Warren SE, Steinberg SM. Acid-base and electrolyte disturbances in anorexia nervosa. Am J Psychiatry, 136:415–418, 1979.
30. Warren MP, Vande Wiele, RL. Clinical and metabolic features of anorexia nervosa. Am J Obstet Gynecol 117:435–449, 1973.
31. Tuck ML, Sowers JR, Dornfield L, et al. Reductions in plasma catecholamines and blood pressure during weight loss in obese subjects. Acta Endocrinologica 102:252–257, 1983.
32. Wadden TA, Stunkard AJ. Social and psychological consequences of obesity. Ann Int Med 103(6 pt 2):1062–1067, 1985.
33. Stunkard AJ, Rush J. Dieting and depression reexamined: a critical review of reports of untoward responses during weight reduction for obesity. Ann Int Med 81:526–533, 1974.

Chapter 19

The Elderly

Robert S. Eliot

Introduction

Stress may be the spice of life or the kiss of death. This is especially true for the elderly. Aging itself leads to many sources of stress—the loss of sensual acuity, loss of loved ones, decreased mobility—and to these are often added stressful adjustments to ill health, money problems, changes in living arrangements, loss of status, and other changes. Yet the opposite side of the coin—the isolation, monotony of routine, and sense of uselessness experienced by many of the elderly (particularly those institutionalized)—is just as detrimental.

Physicians face the challenge of determining whether emotional states, such as anxiety and depression, are caused by external problems that must be resolved to prevent physical consequences, or whether these states are primarily physiological in nature.

As Ernst Wynder has said, "It should be the function of medicine to have people die young as late as possible." This involves more than maintaining the physical state of the individuals. Physicians and social services must try to help the elderly to cope with their problems without depriving them of their sense of identity, control, and self-esteem.

Most stereotypes are wrong. Retirees, for instance, often report better health after retirement than before, and studies comparing healthy retirees with similar healthy individuals continuing to work have shown that any deterioration in health is due to aging, not to retirement. Most of the elderly (particularly the younger ones) feel their

From: Eliot, RS: *Stress and the Heart: Mechanisms, Measurements and Management.* Mount Kisco, NY, Futura Publishing Company, Inc., © 1988.

incomes are adequate and they are in good contact with their family members. Unfortunately, not all have close relatives remaining. Women now in their 70s or older were at their peak childbearing years during the Depression, and had the lowest fertility rate of any American women to the present; one third have no surviving children.[1]

Health in later years largely depends on good health habits of earlier years, but it has been found that people can change their habits at any age. An exercising senior may achieve greater endurance than he had in his sedentary twenties.[2] Therapy of any sort should not be withheld simply because of a person's age. Each person should be assessed individually, as functional changes do not follow a set pattern or schedule. The range of health is much greater among those in their 70s than among preschoolers.

There are some special considerations, however, that should be kept in mind with elderly patients.

History and Physical Examination

A longer time is required for proper assessment of elderly patients than for other age groups, but unfortunately studies have shown that this group is generally given short shrift. It takes time to cover the patient's longer history, even if irrelevant conditions of early years are skimmed over. Problems of poor eyesight and hearing make communication more difficult. Often the elderly have several health problems and numerous symptoms which must be sorted out. It takes time to identify the major difficulties and to determine what is treatable and what is not, to sort out impairments due to aging from those due to disease processes. Disease symptoms may present somewhat atypically because of the interaction with aging processes, other diseases present, medications used, and the less active or limited lifestyle compared with younger patients.

With regard to the cardiovascular system, the heart valves, the walls of the heart, and the blood vessels tend to thicken and stiffen with age. Vascular elasticity therefore decreases, but as partial compensation, the aorta widens, increasing aortic volume, and atrial size also increases. The effects are reductions in maximum oxygen consumption, exercise heart rate, exercise stroke volume, cardiac output, and the ability to tolerate stresses. Usually systolic blood pressure increases gradually to about age 75 or 80, while diastolic pressure increases to the 60s decade and then may decrease slightly. Although this pattern is found in many

Western societies, it is not normal in all parts of the world. The effects are no less devastating than in other age groups. Indeed, the risk of cardiovascular disease increases continuously at levels above 130/85, and the systolic pressure has been shown to be as significant as the diastolic in increasing risks for stroke and cardiovascular disease. Several studies have shown the benefits of reducing hypertension in the over-60 population. Treatment of mild hypertension as well as more marked forms has decreased the morbidity and mortality of both stroke and myocardial infarction in the elderly.[3]

With aging there is a decreased response to beta sympathetic stimulation, resulting in decreases in heart-rate and vasodilation responsiveness. The ability of cardiac muscle to develop tension is well maintained without a major change in left ventricular function. The increase in arterial stiffness may be the cause of the increase in systolic blood pressure that accompanies aging. This increase is modest in normals at rest, but with exercise there is a notably greater rise in systolic pressure in the aged than in younger individuals. With exercise, there is a greater use of the Frank-Starling mechanism (increased ventricular volume) to compensate for increased workload and the decreased responsiveness of heart rate and vessel dilation. Because of the greater increase in heart volume, cardiac output is maintained at all levels of exercise, despite lesser increases in heart rate and smaller reductions in the impedance of left ventricular ejection. Age changes in the ejection fraction should be kept in mind when identifying and assessing cardiac function.[4]

Cardiac disease is often unrecognized in the elderly. In one study, ischemic heart disease was observed at autopsy in 50% of individuals over 60 who had died of other causes.[5] Elderly persons may not be as sensitive to pain. Therefore, a myocardial infarction may present as sudden dyspnea, pulmonary edema, profound unexplained weakness or in other guises. Angina may not occur from effort in very sedentary persons but rather will accompany hypertension or anemia. It should be remembered that women become more susceptible to cardiovascular disease after menopause, and after age 70 the rate of occurrence for women is the same as for men.[6]

Heart disease, particularly congestive heart failure, is a major cause of death in old age. Frequently brain impairment is linked with it. A Duke University study of volunteers[7] compared those with no heart disease, those with definite and compensated heart disease, and those with definite and decompensated heart disease. The incidence of CNS disorder was much greater in those with decompensated heart disease than in those without heart disease. The incidence was slightly less in the compensated than in the decompensated conditions. It was concluded that some brain impairments in old age may be related to reduced cerebral blood flow. The subjects with compensated heart disease and no brain impairment tended to have relatively high blood pressure; this suggests that in some cases mild hypertension may help to maintain the blood flow to the brain at the expense of the heart. However, control of high blood pressure has been shown to decrease the incidence of stroke.

Pharmacological Treatment

In his review, Ouslander[8] pointed out the difficulties encountered in treating the elderly with drugs. Four-fifths of the elderly have at least one chronic illness and often more. It is not uncommon for them to be taking 6 to 12 medications simultaneously, often prescribed by several different physicians. As might be expected, adverse drug reactions are more common among the elderly than among other patients. For instance, drug-induced illness was reported in 25% of hospitalized patients older than 80 years, as compared to 12% of patients 41 to 50 in the same study. Another survey showed adverse reactions in 12% to 17% of patients 70 to 90 but in only 3% among those 10 to 30 years old.

Psychotropic and cardiovascular medications are responsible for most of the adverse drug reactions in the elderly. The problem relates to drug overdoses as well as drug interactions.[8] The elderly are generally more sensitive to drug effects, so dosages should be minimal to start with and then increased to effective levels. We encountered a case of complete heart block engendered by the small dosage of Tenormin (atenolol) prescribed for glaucoma, although often the elderly are *less* sensitive to beta blockers. Indeed, because of reduced sensitivity to beta blockade among the elderly, vasodilators are more appropriate for treating hypertension in this group.[5]

The elderly patient should be informed about the side effects of each drug prescribed and about possible interactions with other medications and with food. Among the many physiological changes in the aged which can affect drug metabolism are decreased gastric acidity, decreased splanchnic blood flow, decreased intestinal motility, decreased lean body mass, and especially decreased renal function.[9] Use of laxatives, antacids, and aspirin, common among the elderly, also complicates the picture.

While it has been shown that treatment of even mild hypertension in the elderly does decrease morbidity and mortality, certain medications may cause side effects leading to mental confusion, hypotension, and falls. Therefore, the impact on the patient's quality of life should be an important consideration in choosing treatment.[8]

Multiple prescriptions are difficult for older people and minimizing the number can aid proper compliance. Patients also need to know just what each medication is for, how and when it is to be taken, and what is to be done if a dose has been missed. Also, it is important to specify how long the medication is to be used, because patients may not realize a medication is for a limited time and purpose and may continue to use it, possibly to their detriment. It will be easier for patients to follow a schedule that is as simple as possible and tied to normal daily activities. The elimination of childproof caps should be specified when not required.

Exercise

Physical activity is highly desirable in the elderly, as with persons of all ages. Physically active persons show less marked declines in maximum cardiac output and maximum oxygen uptake. Inactivity and deconditioning can cause or exacerbate underlying cardiac disease.[3] Good physical condition is important to enable elderly persons to maintain their independence and control over their own lives. Physical activity has also been shown to decrease anxiety and improve sleep and digestion.[2]

Endurance training of the elderly decreases resting heart rate, increases maximum oxygen consumption, and increases work capacity. Exercises, of course, have to be tempered by the individual's capabilities; goals should be modest and increased very gradually. For instance, following myocardial infarction, a patient might walk just one block each day until this could be accomplished without pain, breathlessness, or exercise fatigue. Then two blocks might be attempted. For those who are not ambulatory, arm exercises can be substituted; for example, conducting recorded symphonies is an excellent exercise. Aquatic exercises are often easier for persons with limited motion and can help to increase their range of motion. Warm-ups and cool-downs are essential and should not be neglected. With increasing age, a longer time is needed after exercise for the heart rate to return to normal.

Even modest improvements in abilities can make a marked difference. For instance, exercises that improve a stroke patient's ability to dress or go to the bathroom can improve self-image and may even make the difference between being able to live independently and entering a nursing home. Harris points out that "urinary incontinence may be more closely related to the distance between the individual and his bathroom than to the degree of his bladder or prostate problem."[2]

With appropriate exercises, endurance, flexibility, and strength can all be enhanced.

Diet

Isolated individuals and those overcome by bereavement or other psychosocial problems may not eat properly and may be undernourished. Those in the hospital or institutionalized also may eat poorly because they do not like the food. Additionally, changes in the sense of taste and problems with dentures may reduce eating enjoyment. As a result, protein-calorie malnutrition is not uncommon in elderly patients.[10] Individuals, living independently, with limited transportation may need help such as "Meals on Wheels" to maintain proper diet.

A careful history including such questions as "What did you eat for dinner yesterday?" is necessary to determine the adequacy of the diet of elderly patients. Sometimes they will not admit to an inadequate diet because of pride, and verification by a relative may be necessary. Monotony of diet may also be the cause of a deficiency in some nutrients.

We know very little about the nutrient needs of the elderly. The recommended dietary allowances (RDAs) are based largely on extrapolation from the values determined for young adults. A study in New Jersey reported that older persons living at home frequently had low blood levels of vitamin C, folate, and vitamin B_{12}; those in nursing homes often had low blood levels of niacin and vitamin B_6.[11] Low intakes of iron and calcium have been reported in several studies. Malabsorption as well as reduced intake may be involved. Supplementation may not always improve the health status. However, in the presence of stress or infections, nutritional deficiency can lower the threshold for more serious consequences. For instance, thiamine deficiency, in association with fever can precipitate Wernicke's encephalopathy or acute confusional states. Calcium supplementation to prevent osteoporosis is now generally recommended for all elderly women and men. Vitamin D may also be required, especially for those unable to go outdoors regularly.[11]

Thirst responses tend to be impaired with increasing age, and the elderly may not drink enough fluids. Fluids are important for utilizing other nutrients and also help to prevent constipation, a common problem of the elderly. The importance of drinking plenty of fluids should be emphasized especially to patients with impaired renal function and to those taking diuretics.[10]

Diet prescriptions should take into consideration the availability to the patient of any special items and the patient's limitations because of dentures, digestive problems, medications, etc. Overweight in the cohort over 60 seems to have less prognostic significance than in the 40 to 60 age group, so balanced nutrition should be the goal, rather than weight loss. The older person is more apt to have adverse effects from undernutrition. Modest weight loss, however, which can be easily achieved by moderate dietary means together with increased activity, can be effective in lowering blood pressure, serum triglycerides, and blood glucose, and may even have beneficial effects on respiratory insufficiency and the milder cases of diabetes.

Behavior Modification

Behavioral changes can be achieved with older persons as well as younger ones. Indeed, considering the many changes—in living style, physical abilities, family support, etc.—to which the elderly must adapt, they either must be able to cope or will need behavioral counseling to learn how. Actually, the elimination of alcohol abuse, for instance, is more often successful in aged persons than in the young.

Be Part of the Cure Not the Problem

Too often, physicians see older persons as less valuable, less curable than their younger patients. Perhaps such physicians visualize sick older individuals as on a path to death, and consider it an affront to the physician's art or perhaps it is a reminder of their own mortality. The elderly need compassionate health care that is primarily concerned with preserving their capabilities and quality of life as long as possible.

Psychotropic drugs are frequently overprescribed for the elderly, particularly those in nursing homes. In some cases, the use seems to be more for the convenience of the staff than the good of the patients. These can add to mental problems instead of eliminating them and complicate physical ailments as well. Bed rest should not be so routinely suggested either. It can lead to depression and greater deconditioning that is then even more debilitating and difficult to overcome.

Sexuality, a sensitive area in any case, seems particularly difficult for physicians to deal with in regard to the elderly. The sexual urges and abilities do not routinely disappear with age and the interest and capability has been demonstrated in even the very old. Persons over 70 grew up in a less permissive era and are not likely to introduce the subject, yet it is a common source of concern to them. They need assurance that they are not "dirty old men or women" and that despite the longer time required for arousal, sexual functioning can persist and be rewarding for many older individuals. Unfortunately, institutionalized individuals rarely have the privacy necessary for this important part of life.

The majority of "senior citizens" live in the community and only a small minority are in custodial care. The physician can help older people maintain their independence by encouraging healthful lifestyles and by making them aware of various devices that can compensate for diminishing abilities. Magnifying glasses to aid reading, grab-bars in the bathroom, devices to aid reaching high shelves, putting on stockings, turning door handles, etc. are available and can make a great deal of difference to the elderly. Various social agencies and support groups can also aid patients with special problems. Since self-esteem is based on how one is treated by others as well as one's own self-evaluation, a physician who treats aged patients as worthwhile individuals, deserving of his/her time and care can make a marked difference in their morale and health.

References

1. Rathbone-McCuan E, Hashimi J. Isolated Elders: Health and Social Intervention. Aspen Systems Corporation, Rockville, Md., 1982, p 29.
2. Harris R. Exercise and physical fitness for the elderly. In: Reichel W, (ed). Clinical Aspects of Aging, 2nd Ed. Williams & Wilkins, Baltimore, 1983, pp 90–95.
3. Wenger NK. Cardiovascular status: changes with aging. In: Williams TF, (ed). Rehabilitation in the Aging. Raven Press, New York, 1984, pp 1–11.
4. Weinberger MH. Natural history, consequences, and therapeutic philosophy of hypertension in the elderly. Geriatric Med Today 4:81–89, Aug 1985.
5. Weisfeldt ML, Gerstenblith G. Cardiovascular aging and adaptation to disease. In: Hurst JW, (ed). The Heart, 6th ed. McGraw-Hill Book Company, New York, 1985, pp 1403–1411.
6. Wenger NK. Specific cardiac disorders. In: Williams TF, (ed). Rehabilitation in the Aging. Raven Press, New York, 1984, pp 265–282.

7. Geist H. Psychopathology of aging. In: Geist H, (ed). The Psychological Aspects of the Aging Process. Robert E. Krieger Publishing Co., Huntington, N.Y., 1981, pp 106–107.
8. Ouslander JG. Drug therapy in the elderly. Ann Internal Med 95:711–722, 1981.
9. Greenblatt DJ, Sellers EM, Shader RI. Drug disposition in old age. N Engl J Med 306:1081–1088, 1982.
10. Beattie BL, Louie VY. (Chap. 20) Nutrition and health in the elderly. In: Reichel W, (ed). Clinical Aspects of Aging, 2nd Ed. Williams & Wilkins, Baltimore, 1983, pp 248–270.
11. Munro, HN. Nutritional requirements in the elderly. Hospital Practice, 17:143–154, 1982.

Chapter 20

Drug Overuse and Addictive Behavior

Robert S. Eliot

Introduction

The adverse effects of alcohol on the heart and cardiovascular system have been known for a long time. The effects of other addictive substances, such as cocaine, are less well known but are becoming a matter of concern with the increasing prevalence of drug abuse.

Cardiovascular Effects

Alcohol

Alcohol consumption has been correlated with hypertension—the greater the intake the higher the blood pressure. The prevalence among those imbibing six or seven drinks per day is double that among non-drinkers. Alcohol intake of three or more drinks daily has been estimated to account for 5% to 7% of hypertension in various groups studied.[1]

Despite the hypertension, drinkers may have a lower risk of coronary artery disease.[2] However, they are more subject to various other cardiac disorders. Cardiomyopathy caused by alcohol ingestion can progress to heart failure, and then the prognosis, even with treatment, is

From: Eliot, RS: *Stress and the Heart: Mechanisms, Measurements and Management.* Mount Kisco, NY, Futura Publishing Company, Inc., © 1988.

poor unless the patient becomes abstinent. Arrhythmias are also found in relation to alcoholism. Sudden deaths occurring among drinkers may be the result of a reduced threshold for ventricular fibrillation.[3] Arrhythmias can be precipitated by alcohol ingestion in the absence of any pathology in chronic drinkers but is more apt to occur in the presence of heart disease.[4] Life expectancy of the alcoholic is about 15 years less than that of the general population. Cirrhosis, pancreatitis, and infections are more common among alcoholics than in the general population, but the main causes of death are heart disease, cancer, accidents, and suicide.[5]

Overt cardiomyopathy is rare in patients with alcoholic cirrhosis, and some of these have a less than normal stroke index.[6]

Cocaine

Usually ten years or more of chronic alcohol abuse have occurred before cardiac effects are seen. Conversely, with cocaine usage adverse consequences can be manifested at any time. As might be expected, then, problems arise at a much younger age. Massive doses are not requisite to produce adverse effects, and every route of ingestion, including intranasal, has been related to cardiac problems.[7]

Cocaine abuse has been implicated temporally in anginal attacks, myocardial infarctions, and sudden deaths. Isner et al,[7] in reviewing 26 cases (7 of their own) noted that cocaine produced adverse effects in the absence of underlying heart disease and in the absence of predisposition to coronary spasm. They postulate that the effects are the result of blocked uptake of norepinephrine resulting in vasoconstriction of medium-sized coronary arteries. This in turn causes sudden increases in myocardial oxygen demand and large surges in arterial blood pressure. Increased thrombosis also seems to be involved. Gordon and Thompson[8] point out that the effects may be due not to cocaine alone but also to interaction with other contaminating or co-used drugs such as amphetamines.

The finding of myocardial contraction bands in 28 of 30 cases of cocaine-associated deaths reviewed by Taxelaar et al[9] suggest that a derangement involving catecholamines may be responsible for the arrhythmias and sudden death associated with cocaine use.

Amphetamines

Amphetamines are often abused by athletes as well as by recreational drug users. The effects are variable depending on dosage, frequency of use, physiological conditions, etc. They tend to increase catecholamine activity and thus place greater stress upon the heart. They may increase systolic and diastolic blood pressure, heart rate, oxygen consumption, plasma free fatty acids, and metabolic rate. Central nervous system effects that users desire are elevation in mood and masking of fatigue, but there are also possible adverse effects of anxiety, agitation, and even delusions. Cardiac arrhythmias, which sometimes occur, can lead to acute cardiac failure, and cerebrovascular hemorrhage is also a danger.[10] Reportedly amphetamines have also been known to cause myocardial contraction-band lesions in users hearts.[9]

Other Drugs

The list of abused substances is long and includes prescription medications and such nondrug substances as glues and solvents as well as the more familiar "recreational" substances of marijuana and heroin.

The risk is greatest for those with preexisting cardiac disease. The increased cardiac work load induced by many of these substances can pose life-threatening dangers. Interactions with each other and/or prescribed medications pose additional hazards.

Marijuana, the most misused substance after alcohol, increases the heart rate,[5] decreases the strength of heart contractions, and decreases oxygen delivery to the heart.

Phencyclidine (PCP) causes overreactivity of both sympathetic and cholinergic systems. Together with the psychological changes, increases in heart rate and blood pressure are observed. This drug is often taken with other substances, often without the knowledge of the user. It can lead to panic attacks and violent behavior.[5]

Arrhythmias are seen in users of heroin or other opiates.[5]

The dangers of these drugs for normal persons mainly pertain to their effects on the central nervous system. Those who take drugs intravenously face the risk of infective endocarditis, particularly with *Staph aureus*, which causes an acute form of the disease.[11]

Who is at Risk

It has been estimated that about 10% of the public overuses alcohol or drugs, and that the percentage is double among hospitalized patients. In the U.S. about 90% of the population have used alcohol at some time. Among those 18 to 25 years old, about 27% use marijuana and/or hashish, and almost 30% sometimes have used stimulants, sedatives, tranquilizers, or analgesics for nonmedical purposes.[12] Nor is the problem confined to the young; there are also many elderly who overuse alcohol or prescription drugs, although they are less apt to be dependent on street drugs than the young.

Not everyone who abuses chemical substances is physiologically addicted—that is, will manifest physical or psychological symptoms on withdrawal. Many are able to cut down or abstain when well motivated, often without outside intervention. Indeed, recreational use of alcohol is practically standard in Western culture, but usage normally peaks during the ages of 16 to 25 and declines thereafter. Those who increase their drinking after 30 are probably at risk of alcoholism.[5] The same pattern is generally seen in the use of other drugs.

Several studies, particularly one of Swedish adoptees, have shown that children of alcoholics inherit a susceptibility to alcoholism.[13] A recent study of adopted drug abusers shows a genetic factor here too. Among the younger persons studied, a significant percentage of first-degree relatives either had alcohol problems or displayed antisocial behavior.[14] Mitral valve prolapse, which also has a genetic component, was found to be more common among a group of substance abusers than in the general population.[15] Genetics is only part of the story, however. Other pertinent influences are cultural, environmental, and psychological. Cadoret[14] reported that family problems, such as divorce or parents' psychiatric problems, also influence drug-taking behavior.

Ethnic influences may combine some cultural and genetic factors. Lanier[16] points out that Orientals tend to drink sparingly, at least partly because they get an adverse reaction to alcohol. He also suggests that after thousands of years of exposure, groups such as Italians and Jews have eliminated those with a high susceptibility to alcoholism by natural selection. On the other hand, Native Americans who have had a relatively short exposure to alcohol have not selected out those with this susceptibility and have a higher rate of risk (but this does not tally with the fact that they share the same type of metabolic peculiarity as the Orientals—the absence of an aldehyde dehydrogenase isoenzyme).[5]

In the United States, high rates of excessive drinking correlate with urban living, Catholic religion or less religiosity, broken home, an alcoholic parent, and late birth position.[17]

Treated addicts or those overusing one substance are at risk of dependency on other substances.

Schuckit[18] classified 577 men entering an alcohol treatment program according to their primary psychiatric diagnoses and then followed up 12 months later. The group classified as primary alcoholics were older, drank less per day, and used fewer drugs than those classed as primary drug abusers or as having antisocial personality disorder. They also tended to have developed their alcohol problems later in life, to be more religious, and to have somewhat fewer social problems as a result of drinking than the drug abusers or antisocial personality disorder patients. Those with primary antisocial personality disorder tended to be less well educated than the others, to have significantly higher levels of antisocial behavior, and to have a higher percentage of alcoholics among their close relatives. During the one-year follow-up after treatment, 35% of the primary alcoholics abstained from alcohol for 300 or more days, and 30% of the other two groups also abstained from alcohol for a comparable period. However, at least half of the latter two groups were still abusing drugs, mainly marijuana, while only a small percentage of the primary alcoholics did so.

Conflicting acculturation is a factor in some cases of drug abuse. Several studies of addict families noted a high percentage of addiction among children of immigrants, even without any previous family history of such behavior.[19]

Although the prevalence of alcoholic drinking is greater among those of higher socioeconomic status and educational levels, compulsive drinking is more often seen among those of lower socioeconomic levels and less education, and mainly affects males.

Identifying Drug Abusers and Alcoholics

Obviously the recent use of drugs or withdrawal after heavy usage can influence the interpretation of a patient's symptoms. Present habits and past addiction also will influence treatment choices. Therefore it is important to include questions about drug usage when taking the patient's history, regardless of whether abuse is suspected. Questions about alcohol, marijuana, and opiate usage can be interspersed with routine questions about smoking habits and coffee drinking. It is often helpful to suggest rather large doses so that patients will be more apt to specify their actual usage.

Most of the users encountered in ordinary medical practices are not obviously "stoned" or dressed as ragged skidrow bums. Most will be indistinguishable from other patients. Some, on their way to serious chemical dependency, may already show subtle signs, such as less care with their personal appearance, problems with work or family, or health complaints such as insomnia. The gradual deterioration of judgment, personality, performance, and health eventually lead to more overt problems in legal, financial, occupational, and social areas of life as well as in physical health.

It has been estimated that 25% of medical and surgical inpatients have alcohol problems. Only a minority, however, have obvious disease related to drinking such as cirrhosis. It is therefore important to take a careful history to determine alcohol usage.[5] Signs of antisocial behavior are considered necessary for a diagnosis of alcoholism but adverse physiological effects may become apparent even in the absence of recognized work or family problems. Among many people diagnosed as being depressed, the depression is secondary to alcohol or drug abuse and disappears without antidepressants when the individuals become abstinent.[18]

The physical examination may give clues to chemical abuse. Look for needle marks from intravenous use, damage to the nasal septum in cocaine sniffers, signs of multiple rib fractures in varying stages of healing from repeated falls, bloodshot eyes, etc. Certain routine laboratory findings may suggest alcoholism: elevated mean corpuscular hemoglobin and volume, increases in liver enzymes, particularly gamma-glutamyl transpeptidase; elevated uric acid; and decreased BUN.[20]

Treatment

Acute crises related to substance abuse are beyond the scope of this book. Complexities of emergency care and pharmacological intervention for withdrawal are discussed in detail by Schuckit.[5]

Therapy for entrenched addiction is difficult and discouraging. But the situation is not hopeless, especially for those whose problem is overuse rather than dependency.

It is important that physician and staff remain nonjudgmental of the patient. If there is (or may be) underlying disease, the emphasis should be on the negative impact of drugs or alcohol. Point out that these substances can interact with prescribed medications, can confuse diagnosis leading to inappropriate treatment, and can add to the complications of the condition.[21]

Alcohol Overuse

For patients who are not alcoholics, the aim of behavioral therapy may be to reduce the level of drinking to a moderate level. Alden[22] described a program for problem drinkers in which participants learned a social drinking style that minimized alcoholic intake—sipping drinks, spacing drinks, interspersing nonalcoholic beverages, ordering mixed drinks—as well as ways to reduce social pressure to drink and ways to modify or avoid situations that lead to overdrinking. Participants monitored their total consumption and peak blood alcohol level for each week of the 12-week program, and endeavored to increase the number of days that they achieved a self-set level. For one group, the program was enriched with sessions on relaxation and other stress-management techniques. The overall success rate at six-month follow-up was 67% for those who completed the programs (57% including dropouts), with a slightly higher success rate for the enriched condition.

In treating institutionalized alcoholics, therapy that included training in social skills and assertiveness was found to be more effective than discussion groups. The behavioral training was done by means of instruction, modeling, behavioral rehearsal, role-playing, and practice in real-life situations. In the year after discharge, the group receiving the behavioral training drank two thirds as much as the control group and had twice as many sober days, although on the days they drank their intake was double that of the control group.[23]

Certain categories of people probably should remain or become abstinent. Those would include persons with an alcohol or drug problem in the past, those who are presently dependent, those with a family history of addiction, and those on medications that can interact with alcohol.[24]

To my knowledge, Alcoholics Anonymous has the best record of helping alcoholics to stop and to remain abstinent. However, the individual must first be motivated to change. Understanding what drives an individual to drink can be a clue to the steps needed for behavioral change. The factors influencing adult drinkers tend to be different from those of adolescents who are at an earlier phase of drinking behavior. Peer pressure, social pressure, imitation, and mood change are significant factors for adolescents. Boredom, depression, reduction of tension, and anger are more apt to lead to drinking in adults.[25]

Other Drugs

It is not uncommon for individuals to abuse several "recreational drugs." "Curing" abuse of one substance, such as heroin, may only lead to greater use of another such as cocaine or alcohol. It may be that a defect in the brain's pain, pleasure, and reward system causes susceptibility to a general pattern of chemical dependency. It is likely, then, that a person having difficulty with one substance will be susceptible to drug abuse with other substances, either later or concurrently.[20]

For example, a study of cocaine use among treated opioid addicts revealed that cocaine use increased from 13% of all subjects at intake to 26% at 2.5-year follow-up. While only 12% of the methadone-treated addicts used opioids, 47% had increased their use of cocaine; and of those on drug-free treatment, 51% increased their use of cocaine. It was conjectured that these individuals had more money for cocaine since they were off heroin, and methadone had the added inducement of modulating the postcocaine "crash" when the two were combined as a "speedball."[26]

The treatment period must be long enough to help the patient through various critical times. Reportedly, craving for cocaine diminishes for two or three weeks after detoxification but then returns very strongly. Unfortunately, this often coincides with the time the addict is released from treatment.

Family Therapy

In some ways the behavioral approach to chemical abuse is similar to that used for cigarette smoking. It is useful to know in what situations the abuse occurs, what triggers the craving, and what alternative behaviors could be substituted. However, there are additional factors that involve the addict's family and associates. Often the ways that those close to the patient adjust to the patient's behavior tend to perpetuate that behavior—their expectations, denial or cover-up, reliance on the patient's dependency, etc. The family or lover or other close associates should be included in the therapy in order to alter the drug-enhancement of the environment.

The dysfunction in the family of origin is found to be a factor in drug abuse in a great many cases. Flanzer (quoted by Brill[27]) described the characteristics as:

1. Poor relationships between the parent and the child of the same sex.
2. Severe marital dysfunction and overinvolvement between the adolescent and one parent.
3. Current or past alcohol or drug abuse by the parents.
4. Dysfunctional family communication and alienation.
5. Problem symptoms in children other than the identified patient.

Drug abusers, even those in their twenties, are more closely involved with their families of origin than normal persons.[19] Apparently the abuser serves a function in the family, which tends to have greater problems or to fall apart whenever the patient takes steps toward independence. The patient may serve as the communication link between the parents or other important family members, may be the scapegoat for family problems, or may enable one parent to have a feeling of power or protectiveness. The addiction cannot be ended until the relationships within the family are changed to release the addict from this role.

Family therapy, while having a primary goal of ending the addiction of the identified patient, also seeks to improve the interactions and parenting skills to prevent other family members from being placed in the same position. Obviously, therapists must be well trained, not only in behavior modification techniques, but in the proper approaches to bring the family into therapy and keep them from dropping out when sensitive areas are broached.

Combinations of family therapy with other techniques can be successful. Adolescents in an inpatient facility were treated with psychoanalytic techniques combined with behavior modification, group therapy, and family counseling. After discharge they were referred to Alcoholics Anonymous or Narcotics Anonymous for posttreatment support. One year after discharge, 65.5% of the group remained abstinent; during the same period, abstinence was achieved by only 14.3% of similar youngsters on the facility's waiting list.[28]

Admittedly, treatment of adult addicts is more difficult and complex because they are subject to greater influence by peers and have probably been entrenched in the drug culture to a greater degree than adolescents. However, those seeking treatment generally have become disillusioned with the drug culture, possibly because they no longer receive much pleasure from drugs and are suffering physical consequences. They then are motivated to change.

If you keep drug abuse in mind during clinical evaluation, you may find the explanation for certain confusing clinical states.

References

1. MacMahon SW. Alcohol and hypertension: implications for prevention and treatment. Ann Intern Med 105:124–125, 1986, (editorial).
2. Klatsky AL, Armstrong MA, Friedman GD. Relations of alcoholic beverage use to subsequent coronary artery disease hospitalization. Am J Cardiol 58:710–714, 1986.
3. Regan TJ. The heart, alcoholism, and nutritional disease. In: Hurst JW, (ed). The Heart, 6th ed. McGraw-Hill, New York, 1986, pp 1446–1451.
4. Greenspon AJ, Schaal SF. The "Holiday Heart": Electrophysiologic studies of alcohol effects in alcoholics. Ann Intern Med 98:135–139, 1983.
5. Schuckit MA. Drug and Alcohol Abuse: a clinical guide to diagnosis and treatment, 2nd Edition. Plenum Press, New York, 1984.
6. Ahmed SS, Howard M, ten Hove W, et al. Cardiac function in alcoholics with cirrhosis: absence of overt cardiomyopathy—myth or fact? JACC 3:696–702, 1984.
7. Isner JM, Estes M III, Thompson PD, et al. Acute cardiac events temporally related to cocaine abuse. N Engl J Med 315:1438–1443, 1986.
8. Gordon NM, Thompson PD. Cardiac complications of recreational cocaine use. Cardiovasc Revs & Reports 8(2):29–32, 1987.
9. Tazelaar HD, Karch SB, Stephens BG, et al. Cocaine and the heart. Hum Pathol 18:195–199, 1987.
10. Lombardo JA. Stimulants and athletic performance (part 1 of 2): amphetamines and caffeine. The Physician and Sports Medicine 14(11):128–142, 1986.
11. Durack DT. Infective and noninfective carditis. Hurst JW, (ed). The Heart, 6th ed. McGraw-Hill, New York, 1986, pp 1130–1157.
12. Kamerow DB, Pincus HA, Macdonald DI. Alcohol abuse, other drug abuse, and mental disorders in medical practice. JAMA 255:2054–2057, 1986.
13. Cloninger CR, Bohman M, Sigvardsson S. Inheritance of alcohol abuse: cross-fostering analysis of adopted men. Arch Gen Psychiatry 38:861–864, 1981.
14. Cadoret RJ, Troughton E, O'Gorman TW, et al. An adoption study of genetic and environmental factors in drug abuse. Arch Gen Psychiatry 43:1131–1136, 1986.
15. Stringer JC, Obeid A, O'Shea E. Mitral valve prolapse and addictions. Am J Cardiol 56:808–809, 1985.
16. Lanier DC. Familial alcoholism. Medical Aspects of Human Sexuality 20(5):19–23, 1986.
17. Ray O. Drugs, Society, and Human Behavior, 2nd Edition. C.V. Mosby Company, St. Louis, 1978.

18. Schuckit MA. The clinical implications of primary diagnostic groups among alcoholics. Arch Gen Psychiatry 42:1043–1049, 1985.
19. Stanton MD, Todd TC, Heard DB, et al. A conceptual model. In: Stanton MD, Todd TC (eds). The Family Therapy of Drug Abuse and Addiction, The Guilford Press, New York, 1982, pp 7–30.
20. Breaking the bondage of chemical dependency. Emergency Med 19(3):23–39, 1987.
21. Zucker DK, Kaufmann MW, Donn R, et al. Substance abuse; guidelines for diagnosis and detoxification. Med Times 115(1):33–41, 1987.
22. Alden L. Preventive strategies in the treatment of alcohol abuse: a review and a proposal. In: Davidson PO, Davidson SM (eds). Behavioral Medicine: Changing Health Lifestyles, Brunner/Mazel, New York, 1980, pp 256–278.
23. Eriksen L, Bjornstad S, Gotestam KG. Social skills training in groups for alcoholics: one-year treatment outcome for groups and individuals. Addict Behav 11:309–329, 1986.
24. Mooney AJ III. Alcohol use. In: Taylor RB, Ureda JR, Denham JW, (eds). Health Promotion: Principles and Clinical Applications, Appleton-Century-Crofts, Norwalk, Conn, 1982, pp 233–258.
25. Engstrom D. A psychological perspective of prevention in alcoholism. In: Matarazzo JD, Weiss SM, Herd JA, et al. (eds). Behavioral Health: a Handbook of Health Enhancement and Disease Prevention, John Wiley & Sons, New York, 1984, pp 1047–1058.
26. Kosten TR, Rounsaville BJ, Kleber HD. A 2.5-year follow-up of cocaine use among treated opioid addicts. Have our treatments helped? Arch Gen Psychiatry 44:281–284, 1987.
27. Brill L. The Clinical Treatment of Substance Abusers. The Free Press, New York, 1981.
28. Grenier C. Treatment effectiveness in an adolescent chemical dependency treatment program: a quasi-experimental design. Int J Addictions 20:381–391, 1985.

INDEX